HEAL YOUR BODY

A Novel-Essay that teaches you
how to EAT and THINK in an
anti inflammatory way, in order to
restore the immune system and
treat degenerative diseases like cancer

GIORGIO BOGONI

WARNING

This publication cannot be understood in any way as a therapeutic advice since the author is not legally authorized for suggesting therapies. The author therefore declines any responsibility for the use of the self-managed scientific information contained in this text and, by law; he invites you to consult your doctor before undertaking it

INDEX

YOU HAVE CANCER

I had understood it by now, Doctor.

It was the only thing I was able to say.

I had understood it by now: I had cancer.

He stared at me with a paternal look, almost dejected, but from time to time, he was stern and serious.

Look, I will immediately set up a first cycle of therapy.

You should never do everything by yourself, I take care of everything.

You will come to the pavilion next door, every two weeks for 6 times, at 8.00 am, do not eat that day. We will do the blood tests and the treatment; you can go home in the afternoon. Next week is fine?

In addition, while he stressed out the words, like mine path or ours was a familiar road and largely crossed by others, I felt almost wounded in my pride.

Helpless, and faced with illness. Eager to know.

Yes, of course, that is... can you explain to me better, Doctor.

After countless exams, I can only meet you today and you are telling me that I am about to start the chemotherapy... I am disoriented, everything is happening too fast.

Will I recover? And for how long?

He asked me to listen carefully.

Do you remember that pain in your abdomen that you talk to me every time we met? The CT scan showed a lesion in a position where it is impossible to intervene surgically, so we are left only with the chemotherapy and radiotherapy options.

I talked about your case with my colleagues just yesterday and we all agreed to start a chemo cycle. In your folder I can't find a family phone reference, leave me one please? So Thursday, is it okay? Otherwise I do have a free seat also the following Monday.

338.2884255, that's my cousin number; I have no one else left. Thursday, of course, why shouldn't Thursday go well? My Health comes before anything else, any commitment I had for Thursday can definitely wait. However, Doctor, I wanted to know what you would do to me. Will I lose my hair like my friend Walter? And then how long will this therapy last? Will I be cured afterwards?

The game became hard, just like his gaze.

What do you want to know? The name of the drug we will use in your case? Do you want to propose another one? Why don't you listen to me?

I told you we will start with a cycle of 6 therapies, one every two weeks, always on Thursday. I also told you to show up at 8.00 am, what else do you need to know?

I do not have the crystal ball and be able to tell you if you will need more cycles, nor how will your body react to treatment and if we decide to use radiotherapy as well.

You are in good hands, be patient and you will see that everything will be fine.

Yes, I must apologize but the fact is that I knew I had a tumor only 5 minutes ago and now, almost without realizing it, I am already on chemotherapy...

Didn't you tell me you already understood that?

In cases like yours, it is very important to intervene in a timely manner.

Aren't you happy to start your treatment right away?

Public Health works really well, you have no idea how much this brand new drug will cost you and you don't even have to pay for it!

Just a few years ago, people were dying from diseases like yours and you are worried about your hair?

Listen to me, that I see so many cases like yours, so do everything I tell you and you will see that everything will be fine.

Thank you Doctor, excuse me again.

I have not studied like you but, before I leave, let me ask you one last question: if you were in my place now what would you do?

You don't have to do anything.

You just need to come here on Thursday every two weeks and trust the Medicine.

Or maybe you would prefer to see some charlatan, those who end up on TV, or even heal with herbs like did in the Middle Ages?

No, you didn't understand me.

I am asking you: What would you do if you were in my place?

In fact, no, I just don't understand you.

I didn't ask you to do anything at all, beyond being punctual when you come here.

I did not offer you two alternatives to choose from because you wouldn't have the knowledge to do it, so why are you asking me what I would do if I was in your place?

You're right, Doctor, you didn't give me an alternative but I still have an alternative: I could reserve the right to accept or not the chemotherapy you are proposing and being informed about it, or ask for other opinions.

I wish I was asking you if you would do this if you will like me.

The doctor's face lost both at the same time the arrogance and the security. He put down the pen and looked at his patient for a long time. Then he started talking.

THE RESPONSIBILITY OF THE CHANGE

Mr. Mario, my name is George.

Can I call you by your name?

Sure, Doctor.

I mean, that's fine with me, George…

Well Mario, I have to tell you I think I have started on the wrong foot here. Actually, I'm used to receiving patients who are in awe of the oncologist to the point of not even daring to ask any questions; but you just asked me what I would do I was in your place as a man, reminding me of your right to have more information and the sacrosanct possibility of comparing different options.

These are situations that I'm not used to and honestly, I try to avoid them because I fear them.

You must know that, when I flaunt security and detachment, I am only playing my role as a doctor as I was taught at school. Nevertheless, more and more often I ask myself how right it is to use the image of a self-confident doctor in order to ignore the questions of those who rightly believe to be the first person in charge of their own body.

I thank you for these words, George.

I fully understand that many patients prefer to delegate to the doctor every decision for fear of having to confront the moment in which they will have to make a choice of their own, but personally I do not even find it right to leave this Responsibility to you.

You know, in fact the System is structured so that nobody takes the Responsibility, not even the doctor.

There are specific Guidelines that suggest appropriate interventions and provide for the application of certain drugs against a specific diagnosis, and then we compare ourselves between colleagues in order to always choose the "best" cure, the one that would not be disputable even in the unfortunate event that something went wrong.

In this way, the doctor's responsibility is limited to the diagnosis phase and, once the pathology has been established, the choice of treatment is almost determined by a sort of Protocol.

There is therefore a "better" cure for all patients with a certain disease and this is adopted without discussing with the patient the pros and cons of possible alternatives: if the Guidelines suggest chemotherapy for a given tumor, it is not discussed with the patient the alternative of radiotherapy and so giving him a choice.

But why isn't it done?

If the alternatives are equally valid, it would make sense for the patient to express a preference based on the different and possible undesirable effects of the two treatments. For me it would be very annoying a disorder that maybe for someone else would be insignificant, and vice versa.

Missing perhaps the time to devote to each patient?

No, there would be time to evaluate possible alternative therapies during the information interviews.

The truth is the system is structured in the best possible way, to meet the demand of almost all of the patients who are used to delegate to others the search for the solution of their problems: in people's minds the Politics takes care of the Economy, the Police takes care of the Security and the

Medicine takes care of the Health!

I do not find it even so much wrong, after all, you are the doctor and I have come to you so that you can heal me.

Thinking about it, I just wanted to get more information.

Then maybe I even asked a little bit more of humanity in the relationship between us, but I didn't think I would go so far as to become an active part in choosing the cure.

Or perhaps you were implicitly asking that I had your Healing at heart, that I would also address my thoughts outside the scope of the hospital.

It would be understandable, that some Studies seem to have shown that this attitude of the doctor is positively reflected in the percentage of healing of his patients.

But at this point, I want to give you good news: you are the only person in charge of your Health.

And this fact simply because you are the only person responsible for all the other aspects of your Life: for example like that of the economy and also of your security.

Here, with this talk about the Responsibility, I have just returned your Self-Healing Power to you. Are you happy?

Self-Healing? But George what are you talking about?

No, stop for a moment. You are the doctor, and I came to you because I need help to heal myself.

The only help you require is to allow yourself to understand that delegating to others your Healing it means that you put yourself in their hands and you give up your Power.

Every man has his best doctor in himself: you know yourself better than anyone else does and therefore you are the only person who can know which cure is best for you.

The doctors can only support you, presenting you with possible alternatives, but you are the only one in charge of your Health and you have the duty to present yourself to the point of being able to make the informed decisions.

Your Life is at stake and nothing is more precious than that, and you cannot afford to do less than everything that is possible.

No, no, no, I'm the sick person and you're the Doctor, you are the person who have studied Medicine for so many years and you must know the best cure for my disease.

Are you telling me that every cancer patient should take a degree in

Medicine and heal itself?

No, I don't want all this Responsibility.

I only asked you, based on your opinion, if it was appropriate to ask for another opinion in search of possible alternatives and now I hear myself say that I should treat myself!

Mario, personally I don't even think that you should be treated; neither by you nor by others.

Using the term "cure", it seems to me that you are trying to fix a part of you that has failed.

Almost feeling as a victim of defective genes already inherited at birth, from the exposure to pollution, and from the urban stress or simply misfortune. Perhaps even worthy of God's punishment.

In order to undertake this Journey of Healing with me, I must now ask you to also take full Responsibility for the causes of your illness.

Of course, now I learned that I'm the only one in charge of my Health and now I am also Responsible for the fact that I got sick!

Now you want me to believe that the causes of cancer are not the pollutants, stress and the genetic inheritance?

That I was not actually unlucky to be in 40% of the people who get sick during their Lifetime but simply it was my fault?

Mario, for heaven's sake, I have never talked about guilt, nor will you hear me talk about right and wrong.

I'm not even saying that the physical causes of cancer are not the ones you listed.

I'm just asking you to take off the victim's clothes because a victim doesn't have the Power to change things while you are Responsible for changing them.

Your Journey of Healing must be a journey through Change because if you continue to behave as you always have, you will get the same results you have always achieved, and it does not seem that you are so happy with the results achieved with your Health!

You should also know that you could earn a long-term change simply by changing the Beliefs within you and letting external events reflect your inner Change, without raging against cancer as if it was your enemy.

You will have to rely above all on your resources and rely on the first tool of Power, which is Knowledge; only by acting upon it will you be able to make your choices.

I decided to tell you all this simply to put your Health back in your hands when I felt this kind of openness in your talk and I'm glad I did.

Now I am at your disposal for any questions.

Ok, thank you very much but you can understand how confused it is.
In particular, I did not understand anything about this Change that I
should deal with, and then you described it in almost esoteric terms.
Can you please explain it better?

I am pleased to have drawn your attention to the most important aspect.

Think of Life as a Journey during which you move from one place to another, finding yourself in places and situations Perfect for what you are and think at that particular moment in your Life.

You know what I mean? You do not like where you are right now, in this state of illness, right? Your Beliefs of yesterday have brought you here so you can change them and evolve into the new person that you could be tomorrow in a state of Perfect Health.

You mean that if I think I'm healed, then I'll recover?

Unfortunately, it's not that simple.

You have simplified the theory of Positive Thinking that

believes that you can change the Reality by the force of will.

The problem is that the Conscious Mind only controls about 3% of thoughts and, even by filling the memory house with the words "I am cured", you will still have 97% of the brain that works against you because the Unconscious relies on your System of Beliefs containing statements such as "Positive Thinking is the foolishness of the New Age"... do you understand what I meant when I was talking about "changing the Beliefs within you"?

Modifying the Beliefs, it means changing what you are.

But it's early to talk about all this: I have to guide you in the Change towards the Healing by starting from a reality shared by us, otherwise you cannot follow me.

The only thing I want you to keep in mind is that this reference is the concept of your current state of Health, is a useful moment of your Journey which is your Life, something to which you will retroactively attribute a positive meaning.

Something you can choose to change at any time rather than an enemy to fight and fear with.

Remember that the ancient sages explained "what we resist,

resist, always persists": by putting your attention on something, it is actually nourished by your own energy.

You are asking me for a meaningful change of my point of view but, if this thing will cure me, I assure you that I will let myself be guided in this Change.

THE WILL TO BE HEALED

Nothing will heal you, but what I will suggest will allow you to be a new person who is in a state of Perfect Health, however for now your simplification is fine.

I mentioned all this to you because it is really important; you must know that all cancer patients who have shown what we doctors call "spontaneous remission" have passed through a profound Change in the psycho-spiritual sphere and in their diet.

Obviously you also want to be healed, do you really want it?

You're kidding, right?
I want to be healed more than anything else, I fall asleep with this thought and is the first thing that runs my mind when I wake up.

I want to be healed more than anything else, I fall asleep with this thought and is the first thing that runs my mind when I wake up.

I believe you, I'm sure that your Conscious Mind wants to heal but I was referring to the 97% of you that is managed by the Unconscious Mind. Deep down do you really want to heal?

You know, to understand this, I address a single question to my patients and the answer is often a sort of revelation.

Answer without thinking now, with the first thing that comes to your mind: what's the good thing about being sick?

I do not know. What is so positive about having cancer?

Ok, you don't know, let me rephrase the question: if you knew, what would be the positive aspect of your illness?

Well, people finally pay attention to me. You see, George, you must know that I am alone in the World, I have only one cousin left... since I became ill I met other people who share my problems; with Walter we became friends, on Sundays we often go fishing together.

Now do you understand what I mean, Mario?

Your Unconscious Mind, which manages 97% of your Body, is very happy that you got sick and doesn't want you to recover.

Therefore, 97% of your brain stimulates the endocrine system to produce substances that support your cancer, 24 hours a day!

Your Ego is gratified every time you go fishing with Walter, almost the entire part of you doesn't want to be healed just not to lose this friendship and you don't even realize it.

Wow, you have opened my eyes to something that I had never thought about where actually I was involuntarily feeding my illness.

Many researchers claim it is the same mechanism that triggers the disease.

According to them, cancer is a tool to protect themselves from excessive socio-cultural conditioning that has become unsustainable for the person: the disease is developed by the Unconscious Mind because it allows you to free yourself from the pressure of work, as well as from the demands, expectations and attacks of others.

The disease unconsciously solves the needs that cannot be satisfied consciously.

But how can I change the ideas of my Unconscious Mind? How can I replace the Belief "If I am sick I can live without suffering from the loneliness" if my willpower only holds 3% of the Power of my Body?

There are techniques to rewrite the Beliefs deposited in the Unconscious and they go under the name of Energy Psychologies.

The best is known as EFT (Emotional Freedom Techniques) developed by an American, Gary Craig, and spread worldwide. It's a very simple self-help technique that you can learn for yourself just by reading the basics on the Internet. It is a matter of giving instructions to your Unconscious while stressing your Body by tapping with your fingers on the points used also by acupuncture, it is a bit strange like a procedure but extraordinarily effective.

Through the acceptance of the disease, it will lead you to a new state of Health.

Are you telling me that this EFT will allow me to "teach" to my Unconscious that it is not worth staying sick just for the secondary benefit of spending nice fishing days with Walter?
Now I understand what you meant when you said that Knowledge is Power, thank you.

I am pleased to be able to help you and I add a personal

suggestion: in speaking to your Unconscious through EFT, but also as a daily mental setting, always remember the words of Mother Teresa when she declined the invitation to a demonstration "against the war" responding to invite her when they had organized one "in favor of Peace". Similarly, in order to heal you should not have the "fear of death" but rather the "will to live"!

I appreciate the difference, but sometimes I'm worried about my Health to the point of being afraid of dying and the emotional suffering is too strong to philosophize on the meaning that should be given to the terms.

I understand you and I advise you not to let your feelings overwhelm you but to let them go, understanding that you "are not" your emotions but "you have them".

The Sedona Method by Hale Dwoskin uses precisely the approach of letting go of the emotional charge but you, being Responsible for your Healing Path but also of your Happiness, can do a lot even with simple tricks that help you to not identify yourself with your sensations: you can create separation even by writing them on a sheet of paper and avoid feeling tormented all day by dedicating a particular time of day where you experience... suffering and despair!

I am beginning to change my way of seeing things.
Now could you explain to me something about my illness?

Before going into the more technical aspects there is another important thing, you need to know: never refer to the illness that characterizes this moment of your Life as "your" disease.

In doing so, your Ego tends to recognize the disease as part of its identity; at this point it will be much more difficult for you to let it go because the Ego will seem to lose a part of itself, something that it used to define itself (often as a victim) in the eyes of others.

I have always believed that words have a Creative Power. The Gospels suggest it when it refers to "Thoughts, Words, Works and Omissions" as the means by which the man can modify his own Reality.

Reality is a pure potentiality, we choose what it will manifest.

In particular, as far as the Power of Words is concerned, I

advise you to know more about Logosynthesis, a technique developed by a Dutch psychotherapist, Dr. Willem Lammers.

It allows us to dissolve the limiting energy structures that we have built through our experiences, it is absolutely amazing.

I don't know what you're talking about, but it seems obvious to me that I have to be careful with what I say.

Perhaps it is best that I limit myself to just listen to you...

CANCER AND TUMORS

Very well, of all this introduction I want you to keep the concept that Life is a continuous evolution and that the illness that afflicts you is simply part of it, accepting it responsibly you can choose to let it go because you have understood the meaning.

Now I will teach you in the simplest way how your Body works so that you can understand why you got sick, then your common sense will be the guide that will allow you to decide how to behave in order to heal.

I beg you to use the terms that I can understand, I feel that this is an important step.

It is important and at the same time extremely simple, like any great Truth.

Cancer is usually defined as a vast set of over 150 different diseases that have in common an abnormal cellular development that invades the tissues, but this definition is misleading because it deliberately confuses cancer and tumor.

Cancer is a disease developed by an incorrect Lifestyle in which one's body is exposed to toxins and deprived of necessary nutrients; otherwise, a tumor is simply an uncontrolled cellular development symptom of cancer.

So I have cancer and I noticed it because I developed a leiomyosarcoma in the abdomen?

Exactly, all the tests we submitted you to were done just to give a name to the tumor - a name that, although resounding, only tells you where the tumor mass developed.

Medicine impresses the patient with the diagnosis that are nothing more than simple labels, for example when the doctor discovers that you have otitis he has done nothing but give a name to what you already knew before going to him: "Ot" means ear and "itis" inflammation ... your ear hurts because it is inflamed.

In the case of tumors, the first part of the name usually indicates where the tumor is, while the second is "carcinoma" if developed from an organ and "sarcoma" if developed from the connective tissue, then you have a "lymphoma" if the disease it is from the lymphatic system, a "melanoma" if it affects the skin and "leukemia" if it is from the blood system. With a few exceptions, that's all.

But back to the cancer, we said that the tumor is just a symptom, the warning light that lights up to tell you that you are mistreating your body.

Cancer is simply a state of imbalance in the body in which the internal systems, overloaded with toxins and free of nutrients, can no longer keep cells healthy.

Wait George, you have neglected all about the genetic aspect... about the inheritance a lot of them has been demonstrated.

The existence of a hereditary predisposition does not contradict the definition I just told you: the state of imbalance that I have defined as "cancer" will more easily manifest one or more tumors if the genetic heritage is less able to correct an abnormal cellular reproduction.

In other words, we could say that any genes that predispose to the development of a tumor is a kind of a bomb triggered in the body but it is actually the Lifestyle to light the fuse.

In this regard, you should know that the mental attitude is an even more important predisposition factor; the Epigenetic Studies done by Dr. Bruce Lipton have highlighted how the Beliefs in our Unconscious are responsible for whether the genes play an active role or not and even they seem to be able to modify them!

It is now widely believed among researchers that the Mind of man can change both the genes and their neural connections.

Therefore, I was saying, cancer is a state of profound imbalance in the body and, I add, I believe that tumors are the manifestation through which the body is trying to heal.

This Truth is so great it can be generalized: many diseases are crises of a self-Healing body in which the latter is trying to get rid of metabolic waste through unconventional ways because the excretory systems are clogged.

Are you telling me that I kept a disorderly Lifestyle to the point that my body could no longer get rid of toxins and started accumulating them in a mass in my abdomen?

I am not sure that there was so much intentionality on the

part of your Body in forming leiomyosarcoma, however I would not be surprised.

The Body shows an extraordinary intelligence: have you ever wondered why sometimes a chill causes us a cold and sometimes not? The body reacts to the external agent, in this case the cold, only if it needs a cold to eliminate toxins in the form of mucus and sputum.

But I feed myself with a very healthy and varied diet, I take excellent protein from good beef and I drink milk for the Health of my bones.

I never said that you deliberately mistreated your body with an incorrect diet, unfortunately, you did it without knowing it but we'll talk about that later.

Now I would like to describe in a more detailed way what happened in your Body at the cellular level.

The general state of intoxication and the malnutrition, but often also the emotional state, has exceeded a threshold value that has led to a lack of oxygen to the tissues, thanks to a too high acid body pH.

Body cells use oxygen transported by the blood to produce the energy they need to survive through the process of cellular respiration and, in the absence of this resource, they must choose between dying or finding a new way to produce energy.

Some manage to pass from breathing to fermentation: they produce energy by fermenting sugar (glucose) instead of burning oxygen!

It is this way in which the tissue cells adapt to oxygen deficiency, hypoxia, but this unfortunately tends to stabilize them in an anaerobic state that is difficult to reverse in which they survive without oxygen.

Fascinating, then the mechanism by which tumors develop is so simple! Who discovered it?

But why intoxication reduces the oxygen carried to the tissues? In addition, why don't the cells return to aerobic mode when oxygen becomes available again?

These are the researches for which Dr. Otto Warburg earned the Nobel Prize in 1930.

A body overloaded with too much food and a rich diet in substances that are difficult to assimilate depletes the tissues of oxygen because the metabolism is slowed down.

Think also of the red blood cells involved in transporting food waste rather than oxygen and add the fact that without aerobic respiration the cell no longer generates the carbon dioxide that is needed to extract oxygen from hemoglobin.

And then the fermentation produces the lactic acid, which the liver transforms back into the glucose used by the cell that survives by fermentation, in short, a vicious cycle that often ends with the death of the patient due to cachexia.

Cachexia? What is that?

It is the weakening that literally consumes many cancer patients until death from some kind of infection.

Producing energy at the cellular level through fermentation is much less efficient than doing it through aerobic respiration: in breathing, oxygen allows little glucose to burn and produce a lot of energy but, in fermentation, the glucose is needed 18 times more to produce the same amount of energy in the absence of oxygen.

In practice, the sugars taken by the patient are not sufficient to nourish the voracious tissues of glucose and are less and less so as the number of cancer cells that survive in anaerobic mode increases.

Therefore, the cells, short of energy reserves, weaken and

yield to the pressure of invaders that are always present in the body (viruses, bacteria, parasites and fungi) and the patient often dies because of some infectious disease.

And all this only as a result of eating habits that have clogged intestines, skin, kidneys and liver to the point that the latter could no longer keep the blood clean, accumulating waste on the walls of the veins and arteries until they no longer allow oxygen and nutrients to be absorbed and reach the cells.

Did you ask me why the process is not reversed and the cells do not return to aerobic mode should the oxygen become freely available at the tissues?

Well, within certain limits it is possible for healthy cells to get back on the sick ones. The latter are unlikely to be corrected in the changed genetic heritage but, if their life cycle is restored, they will be eliminated naturally by apoptosis, the programmed cell death.

In fact, this is what all therapies do that tend to bring the body back into balance, but we must see how extensive the tumor is. In fact, anaerobic metabolism is also used by the tumor to grow because the cells deprived of oxygen emit signals that stimulate angiogenesis, the creation of new blood vessels capable of supplying blood, and therefore of nourishing glucose, the peripheral live cells of the cancer.

But if it is known that tumors feed on glucose, why is it not absolutely forbidden for patients to eat anything containing sugar?
Why was I told that I could eat what I wanted?
Perhaps not everyone shares the idea that cancer cells survive by fermenting sugar…

Not everyone shares this idea, however the Truth is that most of my medical colleagues do not think, but merely repeat what they tell them. You will continue to find the sweet biscuits in the breakfast room of the department where you are given your chemotherapy until a directive is issued to prohibit those, even though in the next room the doctors inject radioactive glucose to look for tumors with PET scans.

In practice, we look for tumor masses by observing where the body consumes an abnormal amount of sugar and then we allow patients to directly feed those tumors that we are trying to reduce with drugs!

Wow, you were right: with a few simple bit of knowledge, my common sense allows me to understand what is the best thing to do.

I let you finish the talk but there's a question I wanted to ask you. First, you told me that my body was in a state of intoxication and then developed a tumor to make a small dump of toxins that it could not expel, and then you explained to me how it is the lack of oxygen, a consequence of an intoxicated body, to mutate the cells from healthy to cancerous.

But then why did I get sick?

Mario, first of all, I repeat to you that you didn't get sick when you developed the tumor, you slowly got sick with cancer, which is a gradual imbalance of the body system, and then you noticed it when your cancer manifested a tumor in the abdomen.

As for your question, you must understand that both things are true but they are explanations of what has happened at different levels of interpretation.

Your Body is too intoxicated and therefore, by definition, has cancer. The tumor has developed with the intention of healing, with the same Power of self-Healing that heals a wound, using the physiology that characterizes its current state of imbalance.

It is all so simple and well-designed that, if we can bring

the Body back into balance, the metabolic conditions that support the tumor will also go away, first of all the lack of oxygen to the tissues: in practice, within certain limits, the tumor will disappear like the extinction of the warning light that was warning us of the unbalanced state of the Body!

Now I was thinking that even for the other diseases that afflict Modern Civilization, first of all the cardiovascular ones, the cause is always attributable to the Lifestyle and the Medicine alleviates only the symptoms without even asking us to change your behaviors: we are operated on for a tumor and then we continue to poison ourselves with pesticides, subjecting ourselves to bypass operations and the next day we continue to stuff ourselves with cold cuts…

I was going to talk to you about this, but first I want to summarize with other words how much we said to each other a little while ago because it is important that it's clear to you that cancer is a state of imbalance in the Body that is manifested by developing one or more tumors.

The tumors are formed because the internal imbalance creates the conditions, first of all the lack of oxygenation of the tissues that triggers a cellular degeneration that leads the cells to consume a large amount of sugar.

When the Body is in balance, the Immune System keeps this cellular degeneration under control by promptly eliminating the abnormal cells before they reproduce in an uncontrolled manner.

If, however, we maintain a Lifestyle that weakens the Immune System, the so-called "immune-suppressive" attitudes that we will discuss later, the latter no longer has the strength to control the tissue degeneration and it develops a tumor. .

The tumor is therefore a physiological consequence of the Lifestyle and, at the same time, a useful indicator that warns us that we must change something in our Life.

Healing from cancer therefore simply means restoring and maintaining the Body in balance, otherwise regressing a tumor until it disappears is possible only if, in addition to having removed the imbalance that was the cause, the cellular degeneration has not reached the irreversible proportions.

I thank you for this summary.

I have also understood now that "immuno-suppressive" attitudes are the causes of the development of tumors and that we are talking about the intoxications. Such as from the food, from the exposure of the recognized "carcinogens" chemicals (chemical toxins found in products for the body hygiene and from environmental cleaning but also those released by plastics and asbestos) and, don't forget to mention those, from the emotional toxins such as stress, trauma and depression.

To tell the truth, you were talking about "intoxications and deprivations of the necessary nutrients", but you promised me a subsequent study of malnutrition.

WESTERN MEDICINE

We will have time to investigate every single aspect of it, but now I want to talk to you about what you mentioned, the way in which Medicine works on a patient with a tumor. I will not be critical of Healthcare or of my colleagues because we are offering to the mass of the community exactly what is required of us by almost all the patients who live in fear and do not want to take any Responsibility, but prefer to see themselves victims of genetics and of external agents.

For ninety percent of people like you, the best thing I can do is to take on the role of the Savior, wearing the white coat of Medicine, and prescribe a treatment that does not require any effort, no Change in your way of Life...

Calm down, George, I remind you you're talking to me, that I belong to the ten percent and that is determined to act responsibly and with awareness!

I know that Mario, very well, and you remember that what I'm about to tell you it can only be read on the pages of some books because no doctor would dare to say this to you.

I just wanted to make this assumption because I think it's important, now I'll talk about how Medicine works, as we know it here in the West.

Ideally, the doctor should heal the patient by restoring the state of his Body Health, to his natural physiological balance, so that the symptoms of the imbalance that led the person to consult the Doctor disappear for good.

Simple, right? The Body warns you that something is not working properly by manifesting a symptom and the doctor, through a symptom-based diagnosis, works on the causes and confirms the correctness of his hypothesis when the symptom subsides.

Simple but very difficult to put into practice because Medicine is not up to this task.

To do this the doctor should take care of the patient to the point of knowing his personal history in depth and having the expertise on the functioning of the Body as a whole, but no doctor has it.

In fact, Western Medicine is now fragmented into different specializations, and no doctor has sufficient knowledge, nor the time available, to implement something even remotely resembling to this ideal situation, and so it just turns into a much more modest goal: which is to eliminate the symptom.

Not being able to investigate the causes of the disease, the doctor limits himself to prescribing a drug that reduces the discomfort caused by the symptom. A bit as if the mechanic took off the red warning light that was flashing on the dashboard of your car instead of looking in the engine for the real cause that led to the flashing of that light.

In the vast majority of cases, it is done exactly like this, as well as indiscriminately administering a massive dose of broad-spectrum antibiotics in the hope of killing the bacteria that are supposed to be causing this disease.

This is ninety percent of today's medical practice.

In fact, when I go to the doctor because I have a fever and a stuffy nose, he simply satisfies me by prescribing me drugs that eliminate these two symptoms: an antipyretic to lower the temperature and a nasal spray to breathe better.

If I go back there after a few days because the fever does not pass me then he prescribes a generic antibiotic that destroys everything inside my Body, in the hope of killing the organisms that cause the temperature to rise.

So he usually greets me warmly, recommending me to eat and drink a lot, even if I have no appetite, in order not to weaken me.

Exactly, now I'll explain what was going on inside of you and what you've done by following your doctor's advice.

Your Body has the wonderful ability to heal itself and your Immune System had raised the temperature to fight an infection, to which it had at the same time yielded it in order to expel some waste through the nasal mucus.

The cause of the disease was therefore ultimately only a Body clogged with metabolic waste due to incorrect feeding and the disease was a so-called "self-Healing crisis", a process by which the Body was trying to bring it back in balance.

Instead of being patient that the Healing took its course, you used one medicine to lower the temperature and another to prevent the expulsion of the waste through the mucus.

At this point the body was no longer able to cope with the

infection because of the temperature and it seemed to you "not to heal anymore" to the point of thinking that you should use the antibiotics.

These have wiped out every form of microbial life and the infection has been resolved but it will not work like this for much longer: the indiscriminate use of antibiotics continues to multiply resistant bacterial strains and soon the World will have to face again with an infectious emergency.

What you did was nullify your Body's attempt to expel the food waste and now you are more clogged than before.

To better understand all this I kindly invite you to read the literature of Dr. Arnold Ehret.

In addition, your Body had entered the detoxification phase and intelligently suppressed the appetite stimulus, because when it is busy eliminating the accumulated toxins it does not want to produce others by assimilating new food.

However, you did not listen to it and you ate and drank forcefully, resuming the digestive process resulting in the accumulation of further waste and increasing the aqueous mass of blood in order to make it more difficult for the metabolic cellular products of waste to flow from the lymphatic system to the bloodstream.

And then we should we be surprised by the spread of allergies, asthma and food intolerances even among children? The pediatric practice follows the same guidelines, preventing the expulsion of toxins from the Body from the first years of Life.

And the Body progressively accumulates toxins inside, and getting older, it gets always worse and we find ourselves inexplicably suffering from degenerative diseases, which we dismiss as "characteristics of the third age".

George, but your colleagues are aware of the harm they are causing to their patients by intervening on the symptom without wondering why the Body it is manifesting those symptoms?

My colleagues are absolutely in good faith but it is a question related to the professional training of the medical staff. Let me tell you a little bit of history.

At the beginning of the last century, the main schools of Medicine received the financial support of the wealthy families that were building the nascent market of the pharmacological industry, including the Rockefellers and the Carnegies, in exchange for being able to participate in the educational orientation of these Institutes.

Because of this, from then until today, in the Universities of Medicine has prevailed the ideological approach according to which it is more important to eliminate the symptom with a drug rather than looking for the causes of the disease.

It is the Anglo-Saxon proverb "A pill for every ill", every disease requires the appropriate pill.

Do you get it? This teaches those who follow the academic path to become a doctor for the sole purpose of creating a vast clientele of chronically ill patients to whom they sell drugs for the rest of their lives.

So it is not a sort of worldwide conspiracy that leads so many people to die after a long illness, simply over the years it has consolidated a complex and delicate Business Model that must be protected at any cost because its balance cannot afford any interference from the external.

As usual, the Truth is always the simplest and the most understandable thing: an economic law, dictated by the interests of the drug multinationals.

You're right, it's so simple it's obvious to me too, but I'm equally disgusted with it because I thought that Health should not be subjected to market laws like these.

But in the oncology field there is continuous Research, one does not die of cancer like was used to, because of the progress of Medicine allowing for increasingly effective prevention and treatment.

I am sorry to have to disappoint you, but the publicized successes in prolonging the average life of cancer patients are not as a result of treatments that are more effective, but largely related to the fact that technological advances make it possible to diagnose the cancer earlier.

The rest is all well-coordinated marketing action, and exclusively aimed at raising funds for Research.

The statistics are distorted considering that people survive "five years after the discovery of the tumor" regardless of the fact that they die the next day and they exclude deaths from infections that were a consequence of the disease.

Mario, the Truth is that the success rate of Medicine in oncology is almost identical to 30 years ago!

Moreover, among the staff of hospitals and pharmaceutical companies and all the related industries linked to oncology, are more people living on the cancer market than those that die.

It is an immense business and it can no longer be done

without; today around 40% of the world population develops a tumor in the course of their Life and it is not the interest of anyone who has the power to tell these things to the public, that a cure is found.

We are talking about the most lucrative segment of the Medical Industry where each patient spends an average of 60,000 euros for bottles of chemotherapeutic tablets that cost the Public Health thousands of euros each.

If you have different ideas, it is simply because you have taken that from what the newspapers are writing and you listen to TV and this is simply a part that has interest that you believe those who control Media.

If I find a cure for cancer tomorrow, do you think someone would listen to me?

Or maybe that my treatment would even become available to the public?

If I administered it to my patients I would be excluded from the Register of Physicians and even if I could raise a media fuss to the point of having it evaluated by a commission, you think maybe the results that would then appear in the newspapers could prove me right and put a World Market in my hands?

Do you think they would let me do it? It would be naive of you to think so.

History teaches me that I would have no chance even if thousands of terminally ill patients testified that they were cured: this was the case with René Caisse and his herbal tea, for Harry Hoxsey with his herbal extract and for Dr. Royal Raymond Rife with his electrical machinery.

However, I don't want to be polemic, let's go back to talking about the doctor's approach to the disease and let's apply it in the oncology field.

Do you mean that even the oncologist attacking the symptoms does not try to cure the causes of the disease? Just like a general practitioner?

The oncologist is a doctor, trained by a University, controlled by the Pharmaceutical Companies and therefore does exactly the same thing as his first colleague who treated fever and cold: he intervenes on the symptoms.

Do you remember that I distinguished between the disease, understood as imbalance of the organism (cancer), and its symptoms (the tumor)?

Well, even the oncologist is exclusively concerned about the symptom, the tumor, without bothering to look for the causes so that they can be eliminated.

He also confuses the symptom with the disease claiming "the cancer has spread to the Body and has formed metastases" and "the cancer has recurred years later".

In fact, it would be easier and explainable for him if he understood that cancer is the imbalance that has never been taken care of and therefore it has shown more tumors in various parts of the Body at different times.

In this way he would also find an explanation for the formation of metastases rather than continuing to hypothesize that the malignant cells migrate from one part of the Body to another through the bloodstream, without believing it himself (as evidenced by the fact that the matter does not make a controversial issue of the donation of the blood), and mutate extraordinarily, adapting to the type of cancer that they are going to form (a new growth in an organ would be able to generate a bone tumor instead of an ulcer).

As usual, the simplest explanation is also the most effective one.

Wait, wait, are you now questioning whether the metastases are generated by cancer cells that have detached from the primary tumor and entered in the arterial circulation?

In my opinion, this is proved by the fact that the liver, which filters the blood, is often the site of metastasis.

I have read that the liver is so important that no disease can develop with the liver in good Health: it serves to metabolize fats, synthesize proteins and eliminate toxic substances through bile.

How can you explain it differently?

No researcher has ever found a cancer cell in the blood.

In general I think it is reasonable to suppose that the body develops a tumor where it is weaker; it could be a genetic predisposition or following a greater local intoxication.

I think it's the simplest explanation.

However, on the localization of tumors in the Body, the primary and secondary, I consider the theory of Dr. Ryke Geerd Hamer very interesting; in the context of the conversation we were making, we could say that it defines a kind of weakness "developed following an emotional trauma".

Hamer claims to have found in all clinical cases he analyzed a precise correspondence between the previous experience of a dramatic shock and the subsequent development of the tumor: the location of the tumor is determined by the type of unexpected shock that the person himself is experiencing, the shock is the detonator that triggers the disease.

The whole theory of Hamer deserves attention, according to him the tumor is simply the final phase of a sensible process in which the Body is protecting itself and it is only necessary to let Nature take its course.

Now do you want my personal explanation of why the liver often gets sick after it turns out to have a tumor somewhere else in the Body?

Because you are angry and the liver is the organ connected to the emotion of anger, the millennial Chinese Medicine teaches it and after all, don't we say, "to fret the liver with anger"?

Do not think I'm joking, it is entirely plausible from the biochemical point of view: the liver might just be the preferential target of the hormones produced by the brain when you feel the emotion of anger.

Biochemistry works in this way and through these dynamics supports higher-level concepts such as where the Reality is highly symbolic, especially in the manifestation of diseases.

A good example is the case of that husband who developed a throat tumor after his wife left him with the words "There's nothing more you can tell me!"

Read the Metamedicine by Claudia Rainville and the Verbal Therapy of Gabriella Mereu.

I agree George, your hypothesis is at least as reasonable as the others but this discussion on metastases has distanced us from the discourse we were doing: instead of attacking the tumor, which is only the symptom, Medicine should intervene on the causes of cancer... but what are the causes of this imbalance in the Body?

You have arrived at the heart of the problem, fact is the causes of the imbalance of a System as complex as the human Body can be many.

And what is worse is that every patient has a personal set of causes that led to the imbalance that we call cancer.

Therefore, Medicine does not even dare to enter into a process that, by not being standardized, is wrongly defined as unscientific.

The basic idea is the concept of "repairing what is broken" but, to do this, we need a diagnostic phase that is too personalized for today's hospital standards.

Let me explain you with an example: if Mr. A no longer has the Body in balance due to lack of a certain vitamin and Mr. B has a mercury poisoning, I will not heal anyone if I follow a detoxifying therapy at Mr. A and start administering vitamins to Mr. B!

Add also, as I said earlier, that the cause is almost never just one, and you have another good reason why doctors does not even dare to look for the causes of cancer but prefers to claim that cancer is the tumor, while admitting that they do not even know why it was developed, and attacking it as best as they can.

Well, that one they can often do it successfully: Walter's paraganglioma has shrunk by a third with two cycles of chemotherapy.

You know Mario; the Truth is that I feel like an actor of a gigantic theatrical work, paid to do its part without believing it, in the eyes of the public that applauds the successes of Medicine.

You and my other patients are the only customers of these Pharmaceutical Companies, who collect the proceeds from the box office of this great farce, and also manage to make you believe that they are treating you!

Now the time has come to talk you about the three tools that Medicine uses to eliminate or reduce the tumors in size: surgery, chemotherapy and radiotherapy.

SURGERY, CHEMOTHERAPY AND RADIOTHERAPY

I hope that, come this far, it will be clear to you that Western Medicine intervenes on the tumor, the symptom of cancer, because it does not know the causes of the disease and therefore cannot work otherwise.

In addition, the tumor has well-defined characteristics and consequently lends itself to the role of an enemy against which we need to attack: the success of the therapy is measured based on how much it has reduced the size of the enemy!

The ability of drugs and radiation to reduce tumors therefore becomes the parameter according to which the new chemotherapeutic drugs and radiotherapies are placed on the World Market or not: they are approved if their effectiveness is demonstrated in the tests by the fact that in the patient who took them the tumor was smaller than the

the patient to whom no treat was given.

Excuse me George, I thought that a new drug is approved if is proved better than the best existing drug on the market, not preferable not to undergo any other treatment.

And then there is another thing that puzzles me: this way of testing new drugs, where it requires that some patients are not actually cured in order to demonstrate the efficacy of a new chemotherapy product…

Things go exactly this way and this allows the Pharmaceutical Companies to always introduce new drugs on the market but, if you will, it is a way of proceeding that makes sense because it allows you to have a large quantity of chemotherapists that work on the basis of different active ingredients. And therefore, if a certain patient does not respond to a certain drug, the doctor can try another.

I said, "try" because the patient believes the doctor knows what he is doing while he is simply trying the drugs that he considers most appropriate and unfortunately, the choice between one and the other is influenced by rather unscientific parameters. Such as the words with which was advertised the drug by the sale representative who met the previous afternoon, or the impact of the marketing from the Pharmaceutical Company that produces it at the seminar where the doctor participated over the weekend or maybe the opinion of the primary expressed a few minutes ago in the cafeteria!

In the patient's head the doctor chooses medicine based on the medical knowledge acquired during the years of study and following a long experience but, in reality, the choices are quite arbitrary and within the limited space left by the reference guidelines for that specific pathology.

Moreover, Medicine is not Physics; it has no certainties but only statistical data.

In Physics, if I drop the pen I'm sure that gravity will make it fall to the ground.

Unlike in Medicine, where the knowledge on the functioning of the human Body are so limited and only relies on statistical data: just by administering Gemcitabine we know that we have about 60% chance that your leiomyosarcoma will respond to treatment.

That's all. And this is only because it has been observed that 6 times out of 10 Gemcitabine reduces leiomyosarcomas and therefore administering it has become a practice, a fact drawn empirically but useful.

Instead, I find your second observation, Mario, more interesting.

The double-blind tests, which allow us to evaluate the effectiveness of new drugs, need half of the patients be given a solution without any active ingredient, in order to have an efficacy reference compared to those who have taken the new active ingredient.

Technically it makes sense, but I understand your astonishment when you have the impression that the patients are used as guinea pigs.

Do you know that this way of testing the effectiveness of a new treatment is the reason why some scientists who invented the so-called "alternative cures" have refused to subject their treatment to the validation of Science? Because they did not find it ethical to deprive half of the patients from the treatment!

I think that it can be called the "human cost" in moving forward the Scientific Method...

However, I was also thinking about something else: do you find it so useless to reduce the size of the tumor?

Could we investigate this aspect before going into the details of the individual techniques?

I'm glad you asked this question, I would have told you about it anyway.

When I described the tumor as a simple indicator that indicates the presence of an imbalance in the Body, I introduced the concept at a first level, in fact, things are slightly more complicated and it is now time to detail them better.

It is correct to define the tumor as a symptom, a manifestation, an indicator of cancer but unfortunately, it is equally true that this manifestation, this cellular degeneration, progressively acquires dimensions such as to be an active part in the imbalance of the Body, which was the cause.

Remember when I mentioned the changes in energy production at the cellular level?

Locally, where the tumor is formed, the tissues also degenerate genetically and the malignant cells refuse to follow the natural life cycle: they are born but do not die, and so they form the tumor mass.

The presence of a foreign mass creates further imbalance in the Body: it uses its energy reserves by consuming many sugars and thus debilitating the rest of the Body, it compromises its pH, and requires the formation of new blood vessels, as well as makes significant changes to hormonal biochemistry… basically, the consequence of an imbalance, with time, becomes a problem in its own right because it reinforces the imbalance itself!

And then, sometimes, the simple presence of the tumor objectively endangers the person's Life because its mass compresses a vital organ, dangerously compromising functionality, or maybe progressively blocking a major blood vessel.

Not to mention the physical and psychological discomfort that some tumors cause: the leiomyosarcoma in your abdomen has already become annoyingly noticeable when you take certain positions and soon psychologically, you could not tolerate its presence anymore.

No, definitely: a tumor is the symptom of cancer but often it also becomes a problem of its own with which we must deal.

And here we come to surgery, chemotherapy and radiotherapy.

Yes, in order: we cut, we poison and we burn!

The three highly toxic and immuno-suppressive

conventional therapies.

Statistically it does not seem that these techniques lengthen the Life of the patient while surely they worsen the quality of Life, however, as I have just said, I consider them very useful for dealing with possible emergency situations and when the tumor has reached dimensions that do not allow for the rebalancing of the Body because of its presence.

If you think about it, it is not so strange because reducing the symptom is also useful in other diseases.

For example, fluidizing the mucus, a symptom of the presence of the disease defined as "the cold", by means of a mucolytic agent such as acetylcysteine, facilitates its elimination from the Body, which ultimately was the form of detoxification required when you are sick.

The important thing is to always have in mind the difference between disease and symptom, in order to intervene in line with what the Body needs, and this should be the doctor's task.

But let's now come to the three famous western oncologic practices, let's start with surgery.

Surgery is certainly the oldest practice, practiced almost unchanged for decades; it is simply a question of removing the tumor in its entirety, so that not even a tumor cell remains able to duplicate itself and reform the mass removed.

Exactly, the fact is that the tumor mass is generated by a tissue of the Body and, as far as you can cut it with a scalpel, there is no certainty of having removed all of the volume because the surgeon must decide arbitrarily where it considers that it ends and many times it is not at all that obvious.

Furthermore, if we consider that the theory of metastases generated by malignant cells being detached from the main tumor to be the right one, then the surgery, such as a biopsy, subjects the patient to the potential dispersion of thousands of tumor cells.

Is this why Walter did some chemotherapy cycles after surgery?

It is now common practice to usually follow the operation with chemotherapy or radiation therapy because it is assumed that the tumor is never sufficiently circumscribed to the point of thinking that it was removed completely.
It is almost thought to be able to use a poison or burning rays "for preventive purposes"!

Poison?

Chemotherapeutic drugs are among the most powerful poisons known to man, so much so that they must be handled and disposed of by medical and paramedical personnel following some special safety procedures.

Moreover, they are practically all recognized as powerful carcinogens

The basic assumption that justifies its use is that the cancer cells are weaker than the healthy ones and therefore die before the others. In fact, they are mainly the cells that reproduce faster that make the most of them because this is the maximum "selective cytotoxicity" that all the different chemotherapeutic active ingredients can offer. For sure, the cancer cells will suffer from this but also those of bone marrow and those of hair.

In search of a result, we then try to reduce the tumor mass by administering what is called "sub lethal dose": the maximum the patient is able to take without dying.

This is why blood tests are performed before any chemotherapy, simply to assess whether or not the Body is in a position to endure another dose of poison.

The euphemistic phrase "Exams are good, and therapy can

follow," means, "We believe you can withstand more poison, and now we try it".

Chemotherapy is an absurd practice: in an attempt to destroy the symptom (the tumor), the disease is aggravated (cancer, the imbalance of the Body).

In fact the cells of the Immune System are among the first to be destroyed and this triggers a series of further imbalances in all the Body Systems; furthermore, the Body is forced to use the resources it already lacks to neutralize the poison in the bloodstream, making cancer recovery less and less likely.

Have you ever asked yourself why the Body reacts with nausea, vomiting and a whole series of otherwise characteristic effects of poisonings?

Do you mean that the doctor is killing the patient in perfectly good faith?

Nevertheless, in so many years of chemotherapy used all over the World how is it possible that nobody raises any objection?

As I explained to you, chemotherapy drugs are very expensive and the Pharmaceutical Companies must protect their profitability at all costs, using the control that they have over the Medical System.

Moreover, the damage caused by these drugs is easily concealable because they actually reduce the volume of the tumor and most patients killed by chemotherapy are not shown to the people. When the patient dies of any infection or due to debilitation, following the destruction of its Immune System, the statistics count it, for example, like a pneumonia death because, ultimately, he died of pneumonia!

Of course, it happens that some patient dies of an overdose right during the administration of the drug but even in this case my colleague will believe in any way "that the disease was too advanced and it has taken over, although he did everything he could and he had identified the correct chemotherapy, as demonstrated by the fact that the tumor was responding because it was shrinking ".

However, even the producers of the drug don't want the patient to die, they wish that he survives the massive dose of poison and that the tumor regresses until it disappears; in this way they will praise themselves of having cured him of the cancer and waiting for his Body to manifest a new tumor at some other part, in order to sell him a new dose of poison and hope that he will survive again even this time and remain their loyal customer.

But now, now you're really cynical, you're exaggerating.

I'm sorry, I was carried away by this thing, however things are exactly like that.

As far as radiotherapy is concerned, the situation is no different: even the rays used are carcinogenic and indiscriminately they destroy the sick and healthy tissues.

The effect is probably more localized to the treated part and less profitable business like the first one, but believe me between the machines and the personnel is really remarkable anyway.

Okay, but limiting ourselves to the technical aspect, don't you think there are cases in which it is opportune to use however these techniques?

As I told you, there are cases in which I believe that the reduction in the size of the tumor is absolutely necessary, even being aware that we are intervening only on one symptom.

For very large but well-circumscribed tumors I am in favor

of surgery while I would use chemotherapy only in a very low doses, say a tenth of the usual ones. Instead, I find radiotherapy rarely justifiable: because it exposes to an unreasonable risk in order to obtain a limited effect on the treated area.

A tenth of the dosage? And what effect do you hope to get on the tumor?

As I told you, there are cases in which I believe that the reduction in the size of the tumor is absolutely necessary, even being aware that we are intervening only on one symptom.

For very large but well-circumscribed tumors I am in favor of surgery while I would use chemotherapy only in very low doses, say a tenth of the usual ones. Instead, I find radiotherapy rarely justifiable: because it exposes to an unreasonable risk in order to obtain a limited effect on the treated area.

A tenth of the dosage? And what effect do you hope to get on the tumor?

Obviously, no Pharmaceutical Company has an interest in making known protocols that allow one tenth of their poison to be used, while it has given excellent results by combining a small dose of chemotherapy with other lesser-known methods or special devices.

For example, hyperthermia, by simply heating the area where the tumor is located, weakens the diseased cells before chemotherapy. It weakens them because the heat accelerates the metabolism, in an extremely compressed tissue where the blood vessels are unable to dilate in order to disperse the heat, by starving and drowning them in their own waste. Furthermore, the heat accelerates the reproduction of white blood cells, just like when we have a fever.

It is also clever to administer insulin before a very small dose of chemotherapy: by receiving the insulin, the sugar-starved cancer cells prepared to receive it are instead fed with the medication.

They are techniques practiced in very few hospitals and unknown to the public, the vast majority of structures are under the control of the Medical System, which has no interest in these practices.

Unbelievable.

I still cannot understand how Medicine does not realize that it is acting in the opposite direction: instead of treating cancer by trying to bring the Body back into balance, it unbalances it even more by poisoning it.

The thing is unfortunately not so strange and it is always tied to commercial interests.

Two other cases come to mind in which the Medicine goes in the exact opposite direction to that which would lead to the Healing and this because it always tries to eliminate the symptom and keep the patient a client of the System.

For example, in diabetic adults it is administered insulin to eliminate the symptom, the blood sugar, while the Body has cleverly reduced insulin production because you need more sugar in the blood as it struggles to reach the cells because the blood vessels are clogged with fat. An appropriate diet that has been protracted long enough would cleanse those vessels and heal the patient, but there are strong interests in the insulin trade for diabetics!

In the case of asthma, on the other hand, the Body is intelligently contracting the bronchi so that there is less oxygen in the blood because when there is a shortage of carbon dioxide in the blood, the oxygen is unable to pass from red blood cells to tissues (Verigo-Bohr effect).

Breathing techniques in a paper bag by Dr. Konstantin Buteyko recover from asthma, but there are those who prefer to sell bronchodilators that relieve the symptom and poison the Body.

These things, dear Mario, are very well known but they are written in books that almost nobody reads and the man kept in ignorance becomes a victim of the smart ones who have control of the Mass Information Systems.

As you said, you must responsibly take care of your Health in the first person.

But it is shameful that doctors do not report this information.

Be careful, you have just talked about Responsibility and then you go back to the generic complaint that characterizes the people who feel that they are victims of everything and everyone.

Do you see how easy it is to go back to the thought pattern that they have accustomed us to go?

Don't waste time judging the doctors, they act in good faith, professionally they are grown up believing that they have to prescribe a drug for each symptom and thinking that they would be immediately alerted if a cure for cancer, diabetes or asthma was found.

Even if they questioned each other while listening to us talk, could they expose themselves to the derision of their less intelligent colleagues, perhaps risking their jobs or even being struck off the register?

Do not believe that I'm exaggerating, that all the men of science who have found a cure for any profitable disease have been persecuted, made publicly ridiculous and then isolated; even those who were able to demonstrate the validity of their discovery with thousands of patients cured thanks to them.

Your doctor cannot take this risk, only you can choose for yourself.

It is really true that the Ego likes very much to judge and complain, I was falling back. But now I want to know how I can recover from cancer, you can understand my interest since I am personally involved.

THE CAUSES OF CANCER

Much of what you will have to do in order to heal, well, you will figure it out by yourself, with your common sense, once I have explained to you the causes of cancer.

But before we talk about this, I want to make sure you understand the last step.

Although in some rare cases the reduction in tumor mass may be necessary, often the surgery, chemo and radiotherapy do so at really high price, by aggravating the imbalance of the organism that we have understood to be the disease itself, and where the development of the tumor is only the consequence.

It is sad to say, but cancer is not the enemy: today people die in good part from the treatment.

But let's try to understand something more; I recognize the causes of cancer on three distinct levels: the corporeal, the mental and the spiritual.

This is simply because each of us has a Body, a Mind and a Spirit, and the disease affects the entire person.

On the physical plane, one gets sick because the Body moves away from its natural balance, feeding up with toxins and depriving it of nourishment; this takes place with the support of the Mind, because otherwise no one would get sick; and the whole thing is nothing but the reflection of a process that takes place at the level of the Spirit.

George, by introducing the spiritual aspect you make me skeptical.
I can only believe what I can see, so do not complicate things unnecessarily.

Listen, no one has ever seen an atom yet you don't doubt its existence.

However, even the atom is simply a Model that serves to explain some physical phenomena and, moreover, it is a Model that is updated over time: quantum physics now completed the version you studied in school, characterized by a nucleus with a cloud of electrons, and the Ondulatory Model to explain other phenomena. The same Scientific Reality is less real than you think.

However, if you prefer, I can explain the causes of the

cancer by limiting myself to the levels of the Body and the Mind and then, only later, to give you some ideas on the spiritual side.

I do it because I think they are useful aspects to the path of Healing.

First explain everything in the most scientific way and then do all those nice speeches that I imagine answer the question "Why did it happen to me?"

Well, I can answer that question also by limiting myself to the physical aspect: you got cancer because you mistreated your Mind-Body system, that's all.

Instead of feeding your Mind with thoughts of Love and Joy, you subjected it to emotional toxins, stress, trauma and depression, to the point that all of this compromised your Immune System, exhausted from being permanently in a state of alert where it should "fight or flee".

The whole psychophysiological connection occurs through the hormonal communication between the brain and the Body, the production of cortisol by the brain is only one of the means by which the Mind exercises Power over the Body, for better or for worse.

However, even regarding your Body, you did not treat it better. In order to serve you faithfully it simply needed the nourishment that Nature had supplied you, instead you fed it with unsuitable and intoxicated food, filled with the chemicals that you ate and breathed, like those found in personal hygiene and home cleaning products that you have been absorbed through your skin, and then you exposed it to electromagnetic radiation and radioactivity. In addition, we have someone even enjoying alcohol, tobacco and various recreational drugs.

I'm not surprised that 40% of the population gets cancer; I'm surprised that 60% don't get sick despite this lifestyle!

I can agree on what you say but even my neighbor eats what I eat, uses the same deodorant and the cell phone ... but he doesn't have cancer!

How do you explain this?

He does not have a tumor, maybe he has cancer and it could develop a tumor. It may, as it may never develop, or perhaps not even have cancer.

Each toxin, any nutritional deficiency, everything dangerous to which we are exposed increases the likelihood of contracting cancer. Then you could develop a tumor localized where the Body has a genetic weakness or, like Dr. Hamer explains, symbolically suggested by the brain.

Remember when I told you that the Medicine is not Newton's Physics? There are no certainties but probabilities.

But are there any exams that can tell if you have cancer?

There are risk markers of genetic predisposition to develop certain tumors, but I think they do more harm on the psychological level: when you know you have a genetic weakness for breast cancer what do you do? Even if you are not one of the crazy people who run to have a double mastectomy done, it still triggers harmful mental mechanisms.

In order to evaluate the disease itself, the cancer, perhaps the most sensible measure is the efficiency of the Immune System.

Once I thought that cancer was contracted when the imbalance of the organism was so great that could never be reversed, then I realized that tumors begin to develop in order to be immediately destroyed by the Immune System even before we have noticed their presence. Therefore, I realized that cancer is healed simply by finding the lost balance through the behaviors opposed to those that made us sick in first place.

So it would be correct to say "I have much or little cancer" on the basis of "my Mind-Body system being more or less in balance": the better my balance is the less cancer I have!

And the probability of developing cancer is related to how much cancer I have, localized coherently with a genetic predisposition and with messages sent by the Subconscious that uses the Body in a symbolic way.

So if I were the woman above, who knows that her genes have the predisposition that can easily develop the breast cancer ... well, I would do anything in order to "not have cancer" that is "to have the Body in balance", so that there is nothing to manifest through the symptom of the tumor.

Therefore, I would pay attention above all to what I think and eat, because my every action supports my Immune System or, contrary, the potential disease.

Ultimately then a tumor is the symptom of a compromised Immune System.

Very good, Mario, you understand the concept of cancer as an imbalance of the Body and that of mechanisms called "immuno-suppressive", those that compromise the efficiency of the Immune System and therefore favor the disease.

Furthermore, it is clear to you that in order to avoid the occurrence of a tumor it is sufficient not to have cancer, or to have the Body in balance, independently of what is written in the genes.

All this confirms the fact that it is the Lifestyle that allows or not the genes to express themselves, heredity is a simple risk factor for the development of tumors if you are already suffering from cancer. This concept is well expressed in the epigenetic books of Dr. Lipton.

In principle, however, I could never develop a tumor and have the body in a deep imbalance, right?

Of course, you could have the Body in profound imbalance with a broken Immune System and never develop a tumor, but being into various further immuno-suppressive viral infections. In this case, they would tell you that you have AIDS.

But, by definition, you are not sick with AIDS only if you have the HIV virus in your blood, which is the cause of this disease?

Yes, by definition, but even the fact that HIV is the cause of AIDS is deeply debated; however I don't want to go into that discussion.

Rather, you should know that this also applies to cancer: throughout history, several doctors and researchers have "discovered" the microorganism that is causing it.

Dr. Virginia Livingston attributed the cause of cancer to a bacterium, Progenitor Cryptocides, while Dr. Hulda Clark to an intestinal parasite, Fasciolopsis Buskii, activated by isopropyl alcohol.

Dr. Rife has instead identified a pleomorphic organism associated with cancer: cultivated by the tissue of a woman suffering from breast cancer, he used it to develop the same disease in mice and then found it again in the blood of mice. At the change of the crop, this mutant microorganism is before the virus BX, then the virus BY, then a bacterium and, at the and, a fungus.

These are discoveries that have been less publicized than the HIV virus for AIDS, because Medicine has supported the theory that it imagines cells going crazy for no reason and therefore is not looking for a microorganism responsible for cancer.

I personally believe that these pathogens develop in a compromised environment, but are not the cause of the degeneration of the environment itself; surely, they maintain and reinforce the altered state, but they have not been the factor to trigger the degradation.

However, these discoveries are also very interesting because by killing these invaders, an improvement in the patient's Health is achieved and this is true in many cases.

For example, Dr. Tullio Simoncini claims that the cause of cancer is a fungus, Candida Albicans, when it enters the Body.

According to him, it is the fungus, which in fact is found almost always in the proximity of tumors, to be the first cause, while Medicine claims that the fungus is an opportunistic parasite that was developed there because it has found an already compromised environment.

I do not know if the Progenitor Cryptocides, the Fasciolopsis Buskii, the BX/BY viruses or the Candida Albicans are the causes of cancer or if they simply contribute to supporting the state of disease, but if by eliminating them we obtain an improvement, with the Body returning in balance and tumors that regress... well, you can understand how interesting it is to take into consideration the therapies proposed by the researchers who developed these theories.

But how do we contract these pathogens? Can we try to avoid them? This would be interesting.

Interesting but difficult, because they could also habitually live in our Body and be microzymes, the pleomorphic organisms able to change shape during their life cycle, and so they could hibernate at almost invisible dimensions for a very long time in order to return to being dangerous only when environmental conditions change, that is our physiological parameters change.

However, what matters, as I told you, is that by eliminating them the patient heals, and the Body returns to balance.

For example, the simple administration of sodium bicarbonate, which is an excellent fungicide, eliminates Candida and has healed many people by first restoring the local balance in the tumor tissues, and subsequently the systemic balance of the whole Body.

And do you think that to Dr. Simoncini was attributed a special honor for this discovery?

As thanks he was expelled from the Order of the Doctors because he used a product that was not approved by the Ministry of Health and didn't even go so badly, Dr. Hamer even ended up in jail for healing so many people!

In the same way, there is an antiparasitic therapy conceived by Dr. Clark that uses weak electric currents and plant extracts and also Dr. Rife has developed a machine that kills pathogenic microorganisms by emitting waves in resonance with their characteristic frequency.

Very well Mario, but we were talking about the causes of cancer and not about possible therapies, so let me now talk about the mental aspect.

Did you say that Mind has to give its consent to the disease?

I want to refine the definition I gave you of cancer as an imbalance of the Body by introducing the role of the Mind: personally, I don't think we can get cancer if the Mind doesn't have weakness.

In fact, the physical counterpart of the Mind, the brain, has a remarkable biochemical capacity to rebalance the Body, even if we abuse it.

Unfortunately, the opposite is also true: in many cases, patients are literally killed by a death sentence pronounced by a colleague of mine. At a time when the Mind believes in a phrase such as "Only 3 months of Life remain", because it is said by a person whom the patient trusts, it is immediately and often irreversibly transformed into a Biological Reality.

I read an article that explained how stress is the first cause of death in our Modern Society, even if it is not included in the statistics because its victims die from cardiovascular diseases or cancer.
And it also seems to me to have understood, from what you told me before, that stress inhibits the functionality of the Immune System.

When it is under stress, the Immune System of all animals is suspended in its activities to use all the resources of the Body in facing the emergency of an imminent danger.

The logic of Nature is smart: if a lion chases you threateningly, it doesn't make much sense for your Body to worry about a small bacterial infection in your stomach!

The problem is that today's Lifestyle keeps us under such constant stress, as if the danger were imminent, and this pressure, in the long run, compromises the functionality of our Immune System.

Think about the ways in which the Mass Media make us live in fear through the sensationalist cut with which they propose the news and on how the society and religion wisely cultivate us into sense of guilt for any of our actions or omissions.

Fear and guilt are poisoning our Mind to the point that we no longer even are able to think with our heads and let others choose who our enemies are.

Just in these days I noticed in some magazines advertisements that highlight the text «Seen on TV» to validate the quality of the product, implicitly this sentence shows you that what is said on television is certainly true, good and right.

Precisely, I'm glad you still have a bit of awareness, even if it wasn't enough to keep you from getting sick. I'm sorry.

However, it is precisely through the awareness that one can express one's feelings and, expanding them with imagination, get to overcome the suffering without denying it, but by fully accepting it.

What is this process of acceptance the suffering by means of the imagination?

I believe that imagination does not serve to escape from Reality but to create it.

I will talk about the creative process in a little while, as far as the process of reworking a negative point of view through an imaginary dialogue, I suggest you the literature of Esther and Jerry Hicks, who have been writing books for decades around the evangelical concept "Ask and you shall receive".

The mental re-elaboration allows us to overcome both the emotional suffering generated by the unfulfilled expectations and the suffering that follows the experience of the Body that we call "pain" because, even in the latter case, we can decide to change our point of view and feel good with that pain.

But do you know what is the most important thing to learn on a mental level?

It's Forgiveness, forgiving others and above all forgiving oneself.

On Forgiveness you can read a very interesting article by Larry Nims, creator of the BSFF (an emotional release technique similar to EFT), but the important implication for us is that when we do not forgive ourselves, we are not recognizing who we really are and our Body reacts with the disease.

However, as you can see, here we are moving to the next area, so now you will gladly hear me talk about the spiritual process underlying the disease.

I listen to you, on this aspect I'm just a little biased, but I will listen to you.

As I explained to you, you are a Body, a Mind and a Spirit.

The problem is that your Mind, your Ego or if you prefer your Personality, believes that it is you and that you have a Body for your needs, ignoring the presence of the Spirit.

In particular, the Mind believes to be what it has become in the course of its small Personal Life History, the events that occurred from your birth until today.

All World problems come more or less directly from the fact that we continue to pursue the demands of comfort of the Mind, with its needs for security and reassurance, and the desires of the Body, which tries to repeat the experiences that reminds pleasant things and to move away from those of which it has a negative memory.

We therefore tend to progressively close ourselves in our personal System of Beliefs, gratified by the fact that it makes us feel good, forgetting the existence of the Spirit and living with the Mind engaged in its favorite pastime: by simply judging others and complaining about circumstances.

The good news is that the Spirit exists and that Life is not reduced to trying to repeat the experiences already known to us but, indeed, it starts right where our Comfort Zone ends.

Wonderful, and now that I know that I am also a Spirit, what should I do?

Nothing at all, you are on Earth to "be", not to "do", because you are a "human being", not a "human doing".
I invite you to a Change at the level of your Beliefs, your new behavior will follow accordingly: you will gradually extend your Comfort Zone.

I do not understand to which Change of Beliefs you refer.

Do you remember when I explained to you that even the

description of the atom is only a useful Model for physics to explain some phenomena? And that does not necessarily mean that it corresponds to the ultimate Reality?

Well, give yourself a Spiritual Model useful to feel good, adopt it as a tool to recover from your illness; believe it more and more, starting from your current Belief System.

I suggest the one described in the books of Neale Donald Walsch, he is a contemporary American writer who has written several very useful books on the path of Healing that I propose you to follow.

And what would Walsch advised me to believe in so that I can get better?

In his books, Walsch invites you to be quiet because God loves you, because you are the Son through which he is making an earthly experience and, as there is never any difference between His will and yours, he has no reason to be unhappy with you or punish you.

You just have to try to be and experience yourself as who you really are, the Son of God who has control over the Reality around him.

How is this story that I can create my own Reality?

You create your own Reality, in order, by means of Thoughts, Words and Works... you said it yourself talking about the Creative Power, and you were right.

All religions teach it, you are Catholic and this formula should be familiar to you.

The concept has esoteric roots and was recently explained in an extremely practical way in Rhonda Byrne's bestsellers, which has taken over and simplified the ancient dynamic alchemy readings: the symbolism of the 22 Angels within us that control the Reality outside of us, dates back to the Egyptians and is also found in the 22 major arcana of the Tarot.

The Creative Power of your vision is linked to the fact that God always says yes and therefore your Life manifests itself exactly as you expect it: God transforms your thoughts into events and even the people around you show themselves for how you believe it, because your Unconscious likes to be right and therefore filters your Perception on the basis of your System of Belief. Consequently you believe Reality to be objective but, in fact, you live in a Personal World of yours very little shared with others because you see only the image that you project upon it. We could say that we all see the same World but not in the same way.

In other words, your Life proceeds according to your intentions and, in particular, it is the energy patterns of your feelings that create your Reality and then, by observing your feelings, you can understand what you are creating and, if you don't like it, change your feelings .

Emotional freedom is precisely choosing your own feelings, rather than experiencing them in reaction: by changing your feelings, you change your Life.

Do I really have all this control over the Reality around me?
Shakespeare comes to mind when he claimed that the whole World is a stage and people are the actors.

We all co-create our shared Reality; you can read Gregg Braden to understand how ancient people had already understood the Creative Power to try feelings aligned with their own desires.

One of his books also speaks in particular of the Power of Prayer, I highly recommend it.

But let's get back to Walsch's thought.

In his books, he overturns the usual lamenting of the Mind

by inviting us to see the Perfection in everything, even in the actions of others who, they may seem reprehensible, are in any case aligned with the Belief System of those who put them into practice. And ultimately, there are always useful, because they allow us to know our Truth through experience, in a World where there is no absolute Truth.

Ok, ok, everything is Perfect as it is but it doesn't seem to me because I can't see the Divine Design as a whole, so I can only understand it by looking at the events of my Life after many years ... I have already read this fairy tale!

I remember the story of a Zen monk who professed precisely that there is only "news", not "good news" or "bad news", because we cannot know today what will turn out to be good or bad in the future. All this is very relaxing because then even the disease could turn out to be something good, but at this point what should I do?

First of all, remember that the only reason "to do" is "to be": every action of yours defines you better for what you have chosen to be and this is the only reason to implement it.

You must not cling to the result, even if it is something that today seems to be very important, such as healing from an illness.

Instead, focus your attention on how you experience the disease, without the expectation of Healing, and with the absolute certainty that "the World takes care of you", choosing the events that will prove to be the most useful to you.

Live this experience as a bridge to "the best FutureYou you can imagine," reminding you that you are having this experience together with all the people around you and that everything you think, say and do is a message for them. This is why it is important to live coherently the Truths in which you say believe.

Life is a game we are all playing together and we must play responsibly, as you and I are doing in this dialogue.

But now you're already giving me suggestions on how to behave, while you promised to talk to me about the spiritual causes of cancer.

You are right Mario, but it was necessary to make some assumption and, standing where things are now, it seemed natural to me to help you see some adequate behavioral practice.

I anticipate that what I am about to tell you may seem

strange, but this is a consequence of the fact we are experiencing a historical period in which the spiritual aspect is obscured by the technological development.

You must first know that every important event of your Life, and especially a disease that threatens the Life itself, is nothing more than a request for Change.

I like the image of your Higher Self, perhaps even depicted in the Higher Heaven, watching you walk on the face of the Earth while doing nothing important: study, work, get married, raise children, change cars, have holidays…

George, wait for a moment, did you say "nothing important"?

Precisely, I said "nothing important".

If you think that Life only has to do with these things, I remind you that Life will give you exactly what you expect... only these things!

Including a torn Body, late in Life, as you probably expect it. Someone even went so far as to claim they die only because they believe that they must die, because we have been taught that all human beings are mortal!

But I didn't want to speculate on this, so let me finish.

I said that your Higher Self looks at you, all committed to

following your Mind and your Body, and one day decides to let you move on to the next level, just to make sense of your Life, that you were wasting.

Yes, just like in a video game: by means of a more or less traumatic event, for example an important illness, it invites you to go up a level. To savor the experience of Life with greater depth and awareness.

If you prefer I can give this role to God, it does not matter, but what is certain is that you will be confronted with this test only when you are ready to face it: when the student is ready, the Master arrives.

So be assured that you are ready to face cancer with the tools you already have and that God is continually providing for you, including this dialogue.

On a spiritual level, your illness is a Necessity: the only thing that could happen to you right now.

Well, no. I won't let you slide on this one.
How do you explain to me the very young children with cancer?
What awareness will they ever have from an illness?

I thank you for the question, I would have talked to you really soon anyway of that.

I was explaining to you that the illness is always a Necessity but it does not necessarily have to reflect a need of the patient himself.

To answer your question: a 2-year-old with a brain tumor could meet the need for such an experience by his parents.

Do not rush to judge an event as unfair without knowing anything about the energies that determined it and the consequences that it will have on the future.

But what energies are you raving about?

Have you ever felt the heavy air entering a room?

Have you never thought that what you call "sensations" are nothing more than perceptions with a sort of "sixth sense"?

There are energies unknown to Science just because no measuring instruments have yet been built in order to detect them, energies that the human body is able to perceive.

The Love and hatred you feel determine a field of strength, your expectations vibrate at a certain frequency, the environments preserve the memories of the past and each of us carries with him himself a personal museum of energy structures... we are literally immersed in a large number of fields that influence us deeply.

It is easy to say that these fields exist and that they are unknown because they cannot be measured.
But how can I believe you?

Listen, different types of energies can be measured but technically no energy field really exists.

All fields are just abstractions, useful to explain the physical phenomena.

Let me give you an example: the gravitational field is only a Model that serves to explain the fact that objects attract each other, but has no Reality.

Observing that objects attract each other, scientists invent a field that is useful for them to predict for example the movement of the planets or the time it takes for an apple to fall to the ground.

I am doing the same thing now: observing that you perceive some sensations, I introduce the existence of an energy field in order to explain them.

You don't have to believe me simply because I'm not telling you the field "exists", the fields I'm talking about are just conceptual.

But in particular, which energy fields were you referring to when you gave me the example of the very young child who was ill?

Given that in Energy Medicine the human Body is seen as a set of energy fields interacting with each other and that this energy has been recognized thousands of years ago as Life Force, Chi or Prana; there are also individual, family, folks and whole races of energy fields.

In fact, I believe that every characteristic that determines any subset of the world population has its own characteristic field. Can you feel the historical presence of the field defined by the Jews?

These fields are not conceptually dissimilar from those defined as "pendulums" by the former Russian physicist Vadim Zeland: they are constituted by the energy of the single persons, when oriented in the same direction, and then they live a reality of their own, but without a will.

If you prefer, you might even see them as expressions of the Collective Unconscious expressed in the Archetypes, so dear to Carl Gustav Jung, it makes no difference.

The example of the first child could be the subject of an

interesting analysis through a Family Constellation.

It is a kind of representation, often conducted by a psychologist, during which the participants enter the energy field characterizing a relational situation between people in order to understand it better, but also to solve it. In my opinion, the extraordinary aspect of this one is precisely the therapeutic purpose!

George, I didn't understand anything. What is this Family Constellation?

This is not the appropriate context to go into details but do not be so surprised, Freud argued that we do not live but "we are lived by forces unknown to us."

Read the books by Bert Hellinger, Anne Ancelin Schützenberger and Gérard Athias or maybe have a first-hand experience by participating in a group.

Let's say the child may have been sick in order to allow one of the parents to replicate an experience that had not found the right expression between one of his ancestors.

Something energetically left incomplete in the genealogical family tree and which claimed to find form through a disease.

I know all this seems incredible, for me it has become understandable when it became clear to me that this energetic inheritance is not conceptually dissimilar from the already widely recognized genetic inheritance.

Exclusively limited to the individual, the Nobel Prize winner Dr. Linus Pauling has even developed an energy theory on the causes of cancer, complementary to the viral one.

Damn, I told you that the spiritual aspect would make me skeptical.

It is you that wanted to talk about energy fields; I just wanted you to understand that when God give consents to your decision to develop cancer, doing it by means of Body and Mind, he has absolute confidence in your ability to deal with the disease.

And, I repeat, this has nothing to do with the Healing but rather with the spiritual growth that the experience of this illness offers you, and this is the only goal.

To hear you talk in this way makes me laugh because I am thinking of the fact that the precious diamond is formed from a common piece of coal subjected to the very high pressures deep down in Earth, then perhaps it is true that all the pressure that this disease it is putting on me will make me a better person.

HEALING FROM CANCER

You are already becoming a better person at this very moment.

Now I want to talk to you about the holistic approach with which I suggest you take your Healing Journey.

Once again, I must point out to you that I consider it a Journey "through" psycho-spiritual and physical Healing, rather than "towards" the Healing as intended as an objective.

So far it is important that it is clear to you that your Spirit has given you the opportunity to grow through this disease because it was the best thing for you at this time, having recognized the state of imbalance, the intoxication and deprivation, in which you have brought your Mind-Body system by means of free will that you have.

You must first clarify what you mean by the "holistic approach".

It is a question of considering the Body-Mind-Spirit system as a whole with the help of a single reference guide, capable of understanding its dynamics. Exactly the opposite of what the Medicine does, used to treat different diseases through highly specialized doctors who end up prescribing drugs that compromise the balance of something treated by a colleague... in an endless chain of adjustments. As if we were continuing in the pull on just one side of a blanket that isn't big enough!

I understand, but where do I find such an expert?
And above all, how can I put myself in his hands with confidence?
Every day we hear from cheaters who takes advantage of weakness of sick people.
Moreover, in all likelihood such a figure is not even a doctor, because if he were he could not keep his qualification for very long...

Listen Mario, you have made some reasonable considerations but you still find yourself where those, who benefit from the fact that you live in fear, have placed you.
The news in the newspapers and on TV that talk about unmasked charlatans are widespread just to scare you, I do not say that there are no such characters but you could say

that neither are those that are made public as such: what is spread by the Media is who has an interest in spreading that news and who finance them has nothing to do with the Truth.

You don't need anyone anyway; you have enough ideas that emerged from this dialogue to begin taking information and critically evaluate what you are told by the doctors.

I assure you that, dedicating yourself even part-time, in less than a month you will know more about your illness than your own oncologist. And above all, you will benefit from an open-mindedness that has been precluded to him by the setting of the path course that he followed, and this I can guarantee you will really make a difference.

And if you do choose to be guided by someone to accelerate your growth path because you feel this decision is appropriate... well, my advice is to assess that person for its ability to respond to your expectations: the right person for you may not be for your friend Walter and vice versa. You might need more freedom and maybe Walter more information, or vice versa.

As general advice, I only ask you to beware of those who try to make you a long-term customer by fixing a large number of sessions; I find it right that an expert able to direct you on the right track is valued at least as much as a specialized doctor, but in my view of things, it must limit itself to facilitate your personal growth answering your questions, not replacing your doctor in writing prescriptions and finding solutions.

You could also discover this figure in your pastor or in your elderly neighbor; sometimes the answers are where we never knew where to look for.

All right, once again I'm lost here. Now, you also give me the Responsibility for finding someone who can help me.

I told you the exact opposite: you don't need it.

I invite you only to remain open to the possibility of meeting someone who supports you, by responding to all the doubts that will dwell in your thoughts during this process of Change.

If you decide to undertake an active search for a support person, then this is your choice.

All right, George, all right.

Then since you are here, I want to ask you on what «holistic» principles this «Alternative Medicine» operates and how it can discover the causes of the imbalance of my Body.

"Holistic" is the approach, this does not translate into principles, in order to discover the causes of the imbalance, that apply to all patients, for the simple reason that every patient developed the disease as the end point of an extremely personal journey and there he must proceed in an equally personal way.

And it is precisely on this basis that the Alternative Medicine works, while doctors continue to look for a standardized solution for cancer, a procedure that eradicates the disease from the Body, without asking the reasons why the same Body generated it.

Unlike my colleagues who try to attack the tumor with toxic substances in the hospital, I find it more reasonable to remove the causes that manifested it by aiming for a spontaneous regression.

I thought the spontaneous regression was a miraculous phenomenon, very rare because it was worthy of the intervention of the Virgin Mary!

Nothing further from the Truth.

The spontaneous regressions of tumors are the order of the day, they are simply not advertised because they are often the result of unconventional therapies with which the Medicine prefers not to confront and therefore it chooses to ignore it.

The individual patient's voice has no chance of being amplified by newspapers and TV, subsidized by a Pharmaceutical Industry, which has no interest in spreading these stories. Indeed, on the web are multiplying sites that deliberately discredit therapies that instead have proven to be successful, under the pretext of protecting the population against charlatans.

And, if the tenacity of some patients could find some echo, it will still be liquidated in the usual way: there was a diagnosis error and the person was never ill or the miraculous Healing is to be attributed to previous conventional treatments that have had a delayed effect.

Instead, think of how useful a systematic study of cases with spontaneous regression would be, in order to determine the common matrix and to develop new therapies from these statistical bases... yes, how valuable it would be to study the Placebo effect!

Placebo effect? What is it?

The Placebo effect is when my patient heals for the simple fact that I make him believe that I gave him a very effective medicine, while I only gave him colored water.

Some studies have shown almost identical results between performing a knee surgery and simply doing a mock surgery in which only the skin is affected to make the patient believe that he had been operated... the power of the Mind!

Medicine knows this very well, to the point that it systematically uses it when it has to approve new drugs, but incredibly it does not recognize it as a therapeutic tool, but uses it whenever it suits to explain the effectiveness of some unrecognized therapy.

We are truly willing to believe, and without objecting to anything, to whatever we are told by those who wear the white coat of the doctor, the new priests of the technological age!

Now you're being critical.

Explain to me how it is possible to get an effect out of nothing, I find it amazing.

If you think about it, it really isn't that much: the Placebo, the fake Medicine, activates the Body's self-Healing mechanism by giving the Mind an excuse to give permission to the Body to heal itself. The Mind is blocked by the Belief that the Body can recover from a cold but not from cancer and therefore does not allow the Body to put its natural repair mechanisms in place.

We can say that, by using a Placebo, all the work is done by the system of Beliefs, the Body limits itself to follow the new indications of the Mind and to produce the biochemical result.

In general, any thought pattern sincerely believed for sufficient time modifies the physiology of the brain, which in itself, acts on the Body.

In addition, this also explains how important it is to maintain a positive perception of the events we experience because in fact we do not suffer the consequences of the events in themselves but of the value that we attribute to them, after having filtered them through our personal Belief System.

In this regard, Walter told me that "A Course in Miracles" teaches that things and events have no meaning in themselves.

Thank you for explaining to me how the Placebo effect works, I was starting to believe that it was a trivially way to deceive the patient.

The Reality always manifest what we believe and it is the symbolic mirror of the Mind. We could say that Reality, and therefore illness, are what we think they are.

On a collective level, I also like to think of the World as a set of beliefs currently shared by the population, it is a very powerful image!

Now I want to give you some useful indications to restore the balance of your Body, your Mind and your Spirit; with the hope that you have already changed enough to accept this Reality, I rely on the fact that they may seem to you like a common sense.

It is important that you progressively extend your vision of the World in order to come to accept what today you actually think is impossible, because no intervention can be effective if you don't recognize it, miracles can only happen to those who believe in them!

I am going to offer you a tiring Change in your Lifestyle through new and healthy eating habits, but also behavioral ones and in the way of thinking and seeing the Life.

The goal is that your Unconscious Mind will be soaked and all this becomes your new Reality, without limit yourself to the traditional understanding of the Conscious Mind, and this is possible only through time, repetition and a motivation dictated by inspiration and passion, and not from fear.

The reward for your tenacity will be new eyes through which you will see the World and then you will reach the understanding that the disease was only a means, I assure you that the fact that your Body heals or not will be far less important than what you will realize you have earned.

In short, you are teaching me to Change in order to learn how to live, and not to survive.

I hear you, George, I'm listening.

HOW TO BALANCE THE BODY

I will begin to talk to you about the Body because it has manifested the disease and, by obtaining the first results in terms of Wellness, you will find yourself more motivated to proceed on the path of Change.

A healthy Body regulates and repairs itself.

It hardly ever gets sick and, in such cases, it heals from any disease: this would be the same for a flu, or for a wound and obviously also for all cases of cancer.

It is a fact well known, that in a balanced Body, the Immune System suppresses many cancer cells every day and, to make you understand the extent of this work, just think about when you take drugs to inhibit the functions of the Immune System in order to avoid a rejection of a transplanted organ. A tumor mass can be developed in a few days that normally it would take many years to develop. So, dear Mario, to bring your Body back into balance you simply have to behave according to Nature, with attitudes opposed to those that led you to develop the disease: malnutrition, sedentary life, pollution poisoning and stress.

I remember my grandmother suggesting that I think of my Body as a garden: before planting the seeds and treating them, I would have to clean up the earth from the stones and enrich it with manure.

It is a very beautiful image: removing stones means detoxifying yourself from the substances that have been accumulated in your body and enriching refers to the good nutrition through which you supply the Body with everything it needs.

And all this you can do with proper nutrition, moderate physical activity and a bit of healthy outdoor life.

In fact, nutrition is the main tool you have available to nourish your body but also to help you get rid of the metabolic waste you have accumulated over the years, exercise will help you stimulate your Immune System and your outdoor life will provide you with the sun and oxygen, the vital elements of which you have so long deprived your Body.

But your colleague to whom I asked if I could eat what I wanted told me that my type of sarcoma does not affect the digestive tract and therefore whatever I would have eaten before would have had no effect on the course of the disease.

Now you tell me that a good part of the Body rebalancing work must be done through nutrition... I do not know what to think anymore!

Unfortunately, doctors know absolutely nothing about nutrition simply because they are not taught that during their degree course. I remind you that the subjects being studied were those planned by Pharmaceutical Industries that subsidized schools with interest in selling their drugs, and not to make sure that the patient uses food as medicine.

In fact, asking for food advice from a colleague of mine, in all likelihood you will get the perfect clichés of the type "eat a variety of foods without too much in the way of sugars, fats and fried foods"; words that reflect not a nutritional preparation and spoken by a person who has less culinary experience than the average housewife.

On the other hand, the nutrition plays a fundamental role in restoring your state of Health: it does not cure anything but stimulates the body's ability to heal itself, restoring the correct balance of the organism. We could say that it offers the Body the chance to heal itself.

Moreover, it is indisputable that by properly feeding, the cancer patient improves the quality but also the Life expectancy, for the simple reason that he usually dies weakened by malnutrition or overwhelmed by an infection that was not resolved by an Immune System that was way too weak.

A well-nourished patient has all the resources to better manage the course of his illness and hope for a complete Healing.

You reminded me of the words of Hippocrates, the Greek physician undisputed founder of Medicine, whose most famous statement is "That food is your Medicine".

Hippocrates also taught to treat the person instead of the disease and to make therapeutic decisions giving priority of not harming the organism, I find that they are all words of great wisdom and I am disgusted by the fact that my colleagues do not remember when they prescribe drugs and treatments.

Historically, the change of mentality in the medical field

has followed the concept of a pathogen as an invader from the outside, introduced by Louis Pasteur in the second half of the nineteenth century. It is said that only on his deathbed the great biologist uselessly recognized his error and admitted that the responsible for the disease is always the environment that cultivated it.

Even in the case of cancer, attacking the cancer cells with other toxins, without changing the balance of the Body that have made their development possible, just means securing a future recurrence of the disease with greater violence.

However, if it's all so simple, how come the Medical System does not change?

It's not simple at all; the system is extremely structured and frozen by many economic interests.

Furthermore, the food industry industries, as investing for a long time on the final consumer through increasingly persuasive advertising campaigns, have developed in him a real emotional attachment to the food, together with the use of chemical substances such as the MSG which create a real addiction.

A large part of the population now seems to be "living to

eat" rather than "eating to live".

Some of my patients, to whom I suggested following a healthier diet, replied that they "weren't worth it" because they preferred to live a little less but "enjoying the pleasures of the table".

The Truth is that they consider it a pleasure to abuse with foods unsuitable for the human being and a pain learning to eat properly because they do not have the patience to control themselves in order to appreciate the benefits of what I suggest.

I recognize that the lure of fat and sugar has biological roots, tied to when our ancestors had to take advantage of their rare availability, and that we have been accustomed from childhood to associate it with awards and celebrations, but we must realize that food today kills more than all the drugs put together.

George, don't you think you're exaggerating when you're talking about "foods that are unfit for human consumption"?
Man is an omnivorous animal and I do not see the reason why he should not feed on everything he finds at the supermarket.

Next time you are at the table do an experiment: set it as if you had a guest and in its place put a pot where you will add every course of food that you will eat, put the lid on the pot and heat it all to the temperature of your stomach (37 °C). The next day, smell what you have in your body.

Have you ever wondered why the putrefaction of raw vegetables does not smell? Why does a forest smells good, despite the decaying leaves?

Listen to me, you will understand easily.

First of all, most of what is sold as food, it simply resembles you in appearance but it isn't, because it is very rich in calories but does not provide any nourishment. The processes used to extend the life of the products on the shelves in fact deprive the food from the nutrients, elements and oxygen, because it would accelerate their deterioration.

In fact, foods are deprived of everything that may be of interest to a bacterium or mold so that they are not attacked and they do remain unchanged for as long as possible, but if no microorganism is interested in that product, why do you think that the cells of your Body are?

Do you want a simple and easy rule to remember? If a food does not rot or germinate, throw it!

As for the fact that man is an omnivorous animal, I am sorry to contradict you but simply this is not the case. Man is vegetarian by constitution: he does not have the right teeth to tear the meat that characterizes the carnivores and the length of his digestive tract is that of animals that feed on vegetables, extended to the point that the flesh passing through it has time to putrefy and its toxins to be absorbed by the intestine.

If we observe the gorillas in the forest, identical to us regarding the digestive tract and in perfect Health, we discover that they feed on fruits with a 10-15% of carnivorous contributions and without ever consuming grains, cereals or starchy foods.

Translated to humans this diet would mean 80-85% of raw vegetables, living in a warm climate all year round and exposing themselves to the sun.

Certainly man has in part become accustomed to poor nutrition and he can feed himself for a long time with a little of everything, often without serious consequences. At a certain point, however, the Body can no longer sustain all this, then the intolerances to some foods begin and after that, the diseases "characteristic of old age" take over.

It saddens me enormously to hear that my patients consider a series of small ailments a normal thing; the human body is a perfect machine that should never get sick.

However, it is never too late to start eating properly: almost all of my patients who have definitively overcome an important disease have also become vegetarian and often raw food eaters.

Referring to this last option, I can quote you the words of an apocryphal Gospel: "Do not eat anything that has been destroyed by fire, frost or water, because cooked, frozen or rotten foods will burn, freeze and rot your Bodies".

It occurs to me that last Sunday I noticed a sign at the zoo inviting us not to give our food to the animals, claiming it was toxic for them and I wondered why the chips in my hand should hurt a chimp that is so much like me.

Now I understand that the only difference is that my Body tolerates it better because I used to, even though this one is not a suitable food for me anyway.

Now it seems to me that you are asking me to become a vegetarian while I have always believed that you need the high proteins found in meat.

You, like everyone, have always believed in what was repeated to you long enough in order to become true for you by settling yourself in your Unconscious. It is in fact through the repetition of these messages that the livestock and dairy industry have secured their customers.

I'm not suggesting you to become a vegetarian but a vegan; this also means giving up milk and its derivatives, practically all animal proteins.

The largest study on nutrition called "The China Study", directed by Colin Campbell, probably the most accredited nutritional scholar in the World, leaves no doubt: all diseases are invariably correlated with the consumption of animal proteins.

Cancer, cardio circulatory diseases, diabetes... all we see spreading in the Modern Society is to be attributed to the consumption of animal proteins beyond a certain minimum threshold.

The dangerous substances that the Body covers with mucus or accumulates in the fat to cancel its toxicity... do you understand that obesity is not a problem but the solution adopted by the body to solve the problem? In addition, do you understand how risky it is to quickly dissolve a large amount of body fat that releases accumulated toxins without the excretory systems having time to get rid of them?

Instead, people continue to indiscriminately undergo low-calorie diets that also give them the sensation of hunger, triggering a process that will suggest the Body to accumulate even more fat as soon as they are available again!

You were talking about a minimum amount, so you agree that you need some meat and milk…

No, in good Health your Body can tolerate some meat and milk without getting sick but you don't need it at all: in vegetables there are all the substances necessary for your Body, with the exception of vitamin B12, of which, however you, need very occasionally.

As far as milk and cheese, which I understand you like a lot, you must know that they contain casein, a protein that these studies have shown to be extremely harmful.

But don't expect it to be advertised on TV, given the economic return of the dairy industry and the power it holds over the Media.

Are you telling me that it is wrong even with the fact that milk is good for my bones and prevents osteoporosis?

I don't have to tell you, the scientific Studies prove it: in countries where more milk is consumed, the greater rate of osteoporosis is found. It is a Reality that is little publicized, and easily verifiable by anyone.

It seems that the calcium contained in milk is not absorbed as that contained in vegetables, on the other hand, the casein tends to acidify the Body to the point that the Body in order to maintain the blood pH at 7.35, must neutralize this acidity using the bone calcium and thus making them more fragile.

Some researchers also claim that calcium from blood vessels is also used and that consequently the Body intelligently replaces it with cholesterol... alarming a doctor who will try to lower the value with some medication!

The Truth is, however, that these are only theories because we know very little and the only thing that is certain is that we should never allow ourselves to intervene chemically in order to modify what the Body has decided to correct.

Sorry if I interrupt you but it's not clear to me what you just said about the pH.

The pH is an extremely important physiological parameter, many researchers agree that all degenerative diseases are triggered starting from a Body pH that is too low, or too acidic.

In this regard, you should definitely read the book by dr. Robert O. Young who explains how a too acid pH corrodes the tissues, drastically reducing the oxygen available to the cells through the blood, leading them to death or to mutate their respiration into an anaerobic.

It appears that an increase of only 0.15 in Body pH increases cellular oxygen uptake as much as 60%.

So, summing up your words, we could say that the keys to Wellness are an efficient Immune System, a balanced Body pH and the tissue cells properly oxygenated.
But how can I accomplish all this?

A healthy body needs only moderate and appropriate nourishment and some physical activity carried out in the open air on a daily basis. This allows you to dispose a most of the poisons to which we are inevitably subjected.

If instead the physiology of the Body has degenerated into a state of imbalance, it becomes absolutely necessary to avoid exposure to any toxin, and detoxify those already absorbed by introducing some nutritional corrective actions: nothing in particular, it is simply to enrich the organism with exceptional doses of the substances, which were deprived in order to help it restore its normal vital functions. Once again, my advice is based on simple common sense.

So a healthy Lifestyle is also the basic attitude to adopt if you are already sick, actually, I find it very sensible.
But how can Medicine ignore the role of nutrition in curing cancer?

I suggest changing doctors to every patient who is told that nutrition does not matter, our Body is definitely, what we eat.

As for the attitude of the Medicine... well, I find it really sad: it has come to admit that a diet rich in fruit and vegetables reduces the risk of contracting cancer and leave it there, but it cannot recognize that this food regime also has other therapeutic functions because it must protect the economic interests of drug multinationals.

I noticed even on the sliced apple of McDonalds it is indicated that by eating it you are taking one of the five daily servings of fruit and vegetables recommended in a healthy diet.

Recently it has also returned to talk on TV and newspapers about reducing the meat consumption.

You're right when you claim that, at least in terms of prevention, the indications go in a specific direction, but could you give me some practical advice on what to eat?

I will do it willingly, as long as they do not become a sort of "doctor's orders"; from everything we have said so far, I hope it is clear to you that it would be counterproductive to transform my advice into another medical prescription.

From my point of view the human being should eat almost exclusively raw vegetables, varying from the season but always choosing the better qualities and with a preference for those with more interesting colors because they are richer in nutrients.

In order not to feed the tumor cells and the fungal infections that suppress the Immune System, the cancer patient should refrain from everything that is sugary and therefore limit himself to vegetables.

To complete this diet, I believe only legumes and seeds are

necessary; in particular, those just sprouted because they possess an extraordinary Life force.

For reasons that I do not have time to go into deeper, I do not recommend soy and its derivatives.

As you understand, I like to think we can still enjoy everything we want to eat in a small percentage from our food, a kind of taste gratification we all value.

However, for most of one's diet it is important to stick to what I have just told you, by taking care to replace the widespread mental paradigm of "I want but I cannot" with the much more empowering paradigm of "I can but I don't want".

It must be a search for healthy foods, not a renunciation of harmful ones.

That's all?

Your advice is reduced to eating, mainly and as much as possible raw, vegetables, sprouted legumes, seeds and seasonal fruit?

No indication on the quality and the quantity of the micronutrients?

The whole food, fresh and raw, contains much more than the single substances that we know and, above all, it combines them in synergistic actions still unknown to us.

In other words, Nature has put in an apple completely different bio-available nutrients, useful to the human Body, only some of which are known and whose combined effects we absolutely do not know.

Cooking fruit and vegetables deprives this food of most of the substances useful to our body, first of all the enzymes that are immediately destroyed by light and temperature.

Enzymes are used to digest food and, for this purpose, they are also produced by our Body.

If we eat raw fruits and vegetables, we take enzymes through food and, those not used for digestion, end up directly in the bloodstream and support the functionality of our Immune System, attacking the protein coating of cancer cells that does not allow them to be recognized as a foreign body. It is a theory credited as far back as 1888, at the base of all the Metabolic Therapies that use protein-digestive enzymes.

If otherwise we always eat "dead" food that does not even contain the enzymes to self-digest, the Body must continue to use those produced internally by the pancreas, ending up with its reserves exhausted and then, having terminated these resources, it yields to the onset of diseases caused by the accumulation of undigested proteins.

According to dr. William Donald Kelley and, before him, Dr. John Beard, cancer is a direct consequence of the presence of undigested proteins in the Body that make the lymph less fluid and therefore less able to keep the intercellular space clean from the metabolic waste of the cells.

Think about it, based on these theoretical bases, Dr. Edward Howell defined the amount of enzymes present in the Body as the measure of the person's vital energy.

But then my grandmother was wrong because when I was sick and she gave me to eat only cooked apples!
I needed nourishment because I was in bed and I had to recover from the flu and she gave me something that didn't feed me at all!

No, Mario, your grandmother did very well but you still don't understand it because you continue to believe that the Body needs more food to recover and the exact opposite is true.

Cooked apples do not feed, nor do they provide vitamins, and it is exactly what you need to recover from an illness. A sort of almost fasting.

The acute phases of diseases serve to cleanse the Body of the waste that is accumulated inside, which may be crystalloid (the acids joined to the calcium taken from the bones) or colloidal (such as mucus, phlegm and pus), and therefore they are cured first of all by avoiding to take more food: committing the to Body to digest and metabolize new nutrients means to inhibit the ongoing Healing process.

By forcibly eating and suppressing symptoms with drugs, the Body is prevented from cleaning itself up and consequently the chronic problems such as allergies, bronchitis, asthma, visual and growth disorders develop... and eventually also degenerative diseases such as cancer.

Therefore, the therapeutic fasting is an extremely sensible procedure.

I find fasting to be sensible during the acute phase of a disease but also to be put into practice periodically, perhaps once a week to purify yourself.

Even getting used to eating only once a day makes sense, it's a sort of daily "24-hour fast".

The person in good Health must not worry about eating too little: the Essene Gospel of Peace claimed that the human being needs the amount of food contained in a bowl, roughly corresponding to the capacity of the stomach, and the majority of people in the World does not eat more.

I can only advise you to gradually reduce the amount of food your Body is used to consume: sudden and drastic fasts trigger a purification process that is so violent because it drains a large quantity of toxins into the blood, which the excretory organs, typically liver and kidneys, fail to manage and produce strong illnesses that are mistaken taking for insufficient nutrition.

Furthermore, by starving any parasites present in the Body, one risks that they may feed on the organs that host them, but this is a topic in which I prefer not to go into.

The Truth is that the quantity of food kills at least as much as the poor quality does: in industrialized countries, one gets sick because of the excess of food, and does not die of hunger.

However, in your case as in all patients suffering from degenerative diseases, I do not recommend fasting right away, because you especially need to rebalance your Body and I do not find it appropriate to subject it to the work done by purification and triggered by fasting.

After all, the experience has shown that fasts actually reduce tumors but that they immediately start growing back again as soon as you go back to eating.

Instead, keep the diet without any animal protein as a base, which I recommend to everyone and enrich it with supplements that can make up for all the deficiencies that led to the imbalance.

Then you are in favor of food supplements.
I have heard conflicting opinions on the potential benefits of taking pills and vitamin tablets.

As I explained to you, I believe that a Body in Health and properly fed does not need any integration, at the limit I find it useful to increase the amount of nutrients that are taken simply by eating a greater quantity of fruit and vegetables.

And this can easily be done by turning them into liquid by means of a juicer or a cold squeezer, the latter being preferable as the centrifuge rotor heats up, destroys the enzymes, and incorporates a large quantity of oxygen in the swirling motion, which deteriorates the juice by accelerating the decomposition.

Drinking fruit and vegetable juice instead of eating it also has the advantage of not engaging the Body in the digestive phase, which is always expensive in terms of energy, but of ingesting a food that can be directly assimilated by the intestine.

As I told you, however, you who suffer from cancer need a quantity of nutrients that is far superior and therefore difficult to satisfy with food alone.

Many of my colleagues do not understand that the RDAs, the indications about the quantity of vitamins recommended every day, are valid for a healthy person while the cancer patient needs many times as much.

However, the so-called "therapeutic doses" go even beyond the needs of the patient, because they are administered with the intent to cure.

To give you an example, if it is true that the RDA of vitamin C is 0.06 g/day, it is estimated that the dose needed for a cancer patient undergoing chemotherapy is in the order of 3-5 g/day, while the therapeutic dose could be 10-15 g/day. Before you are impressed by those numbers, you need to know that vitamin C has been shown to have no side effects and is given daily for years in the vein at a dose of 100 g/day!

Do you mean that I can heal by taking vitamin supplements or that cancer is a vitamin deficiency?

Vitamins do not cure your cancer but are necessary to support the Healing force that resides within you, as they are very useful in helping your Body to come back into balance.

As for the fact that cancer is a vitamin deficiency... well, having defined it as a metabolic imbalance of the Body, in some cases it could also be due to a vitamin deficiency, in the hypothesis that vitamins are necessary for the normal cell life cycle that should end with apoptosis, the programmed death.

There are people who believe, based on the Studies of Dr. Ernest T. Krebs, that the cause of cancer is a deficiency of a certain vitamin, B17 (also known as amygdalin or laetrile), and that it can be cured simply by taking it in large quantities.

The thing would not even be so surprising: after all, for decades doctors searched for the virus that killed the sailors who fell ill with scurvy, only to discover that it did not exist because scurvy was the consequence of vitamin C insufficiency, which the sailors were not getting for a long time.

Many people have recovered from cancer and have seen cancers disappear by eating bitter seeds, including the very rich B17 apricot and apple kernels, to the point that Health authorities have bothered to declare this substance illegal, but I do not believe that this treatment can be standardized. In this regard, you can still read the case of Jason Vale and the literature of journalist Edward Griffin.

As I have already told you, the cure of cancer must be individualized by correcting the causes of the imbalance in the patient's Body; for some it may be the lack of a substance, for others it may be the exposure to a toxin.

Yes, you told me. But you also told me that it is not so easy to find out the cause of the organism's imbalance.

In fact, without further study on the individual case, I suggest an intervention with a broad-spectrum of multi-vitamins enriched with mineral salts, lots of vitamin C, coenzyme Q10 and at least selenium and niacin. The beta-carotene I prefer is taken through a considerable consumption of raw carrots.

The antioxidant effects of vitamin C, which is great especially if you are exposed to the oxidizing action of radiotherapy that destroys cells by depriving them of the electrons, is also found in green tea.

Particular attention should then be paid to the "good" omega-3 fatty acids, whose first source is flaxseed oil, combined with the right proteins, but to talk about that I would need to tell you about the books of Dr. Johanna Budwig, so much it is worth referring to her.

In short, these are the general indications about what should never be lacking in the cancer patient in terms of food integration.

Besides, all the nutritional therapies for the treatment of cancer say nothing different: a raw vegetarian base, enriched with specific supplements.

Read the books of Max Gerson and his daughter Charlotte, you will be amazed by the potential of a diet like this, which, among other things, has the power to raise the potassium values by reducing those of sodium, always present in excess in cancer patients and in the average person of this Modern Civilization in general.

It should come as no surprise that Gerson therapy, undertaken for cancer, also often treats diabetes, arthritis and heart disease simultaneously.

Surprisingly the official position of Medicine claims that a diet can improve the Quality of Life and reduce the risk of developing a tumor, but has no therapeutic value.

Do you know that I asked a colleague of yours if food supplements would have been useful to me and he looked at me, as I was stupid?

And I felt so, while I was in awe.

The Pharmaceutical Companies see the supplement market as a competitor and disseminate information in scientific journals so that doctors themselves consider these supplements of no use and consequently they discredit those in the patient's eyes.

The strategy works: just yesterday I heard a patient undergoing chemotherapy being told not to take vitamin C because it would also protect cancer cells from the effects of drugs, while several Studies, starting with the controversial ones of Dr. Pauling, have highlighted how the antioxidant action of vitamin C protects the healthy cells and at the same time carries out a destructive action on diseased cells, because they absorb it in such large quantities by exchanging the molecule for the glucose.

Moreover, it appears that there is already a worldwide legislative project called "Codex Alimentarius" which, with the usual excuse of protecting the population, prohibits the sale of supplements at doses higher than the RDA, thus eliminating any possible therapeutic effect of these ones.

The public enemies of the near future will be the supplements, as today is the sugar. The latter, although it is certainly harmful (it is an addictive drug and activates insulin, the hormone that produces body fat) is still fought without criteria: for example, without reserving the same attention to carbohydrates, which the Body immediately transforms into sugars.

In any case, don't believe the companies that operate in the supplement sector are better than those that share the drug market: I've seen everything sold, and promising miraculous effects, even the freeze-dried vegetables in capsules!

I remember when I was a child cartoons suggesting that the consumption of vegetables gave super-powers: I remember the spinach of Popeye and the Bugs Bunny carrots.

Then something must have changed because cinematography has begun to show the super-powers acquired through radioactivity and genetic mutations, I think of the Fantastic 4 and the Hulk but also of many of the most recent cartoon characters, those who our children watch in front of TV.

Unfortunately, a raw carrot juice does not heal you from cancer, but the mental attitude, which is a part of this, is the most sensible way to take for many patients, rather than being intoxicated with the poisons administered by my colleagues.

Let me tell you a joke about Western Medicine in line with what I've told you so far: just as a cold is not provoked by an aspirin deficiency, in the same way a cancer is not caused to a lack of chemotherapy!

Right reflection, it is not clear why we should heal by adding to our Body something it surely never needed!

Listen, George, I would say we talked enough about the nutrition, but first you also talked about the importance of physical exercise.

Beyond the benefits for the cardiovascular and

musculoskeletal systems, physical exercise is essential for the tissue detoxification.

Surely, you can detoxify yourself through fasting, through a diet based on raw vegetables with a food supplement that reactivates the correct physiology of the Body and the functions of the excretory organs. Or through the much ridiculed coffee enemas for liver cleansing that help to dispose of the toxic waste products from a tumor mass that is dissolving, through therapies aimed at eliminating heavy metals such as the chelating one aimed at cleaning the arteries, through sweating in a sauna or perhaps through the specific actions such as removal of dental amalgam and devitalized teeth... but you cannot neglect the simplest detoxification: that through the physical exercise.

In our Body, the lymphatic system collects all the cellular metabolic waste and discharges it into the blood, which is then regularly cleaned, but what happens if the lymph does not flow?

You can imagine it: the tissues get clogged and gradually you get sick.

And how does the lymph flow in the lymphatic system if the latter is not provided with a pump, just like that of the blood?

Of course, through the movement of your muscles.

Now you understand the need for moderate physical activity to keep the body clean.

Something that goes far beyond having a good tonic look to show off in public, something that has above all a lot to do with your Health.

On the other hand, you don't even have to exaggerate with physical exercise, and I'm not referring to competitive activities in which the repetition of movements gets to consume the cartilaginous structure of the Body, but I want to emphasize the meaning of fatigue that, as you well know, takes over when the muscles begin to produce the lactic acid.

If you remember the importance of maintaining a proper body pH, you will understand the work for rebalancing the pH that you are requesting your Body to do when this acid appears in the musculature but also the resources it will have to consume to put it into action.

The fatigue is telling you to stop the exercise, nothing more simple than that.

Forgive me if I keep asking you for practical examples, but could you tell me a physical activity that is suitable for everyone, able to effectively stimulate a high flow of the lymphatic system, without producing lactic acid in the musculature?

With a minimal expense you can buy a mini trampoline, it is a cloth stretched on a circular metal structure that you find in almost any sporting goods stores.

You can buy the smaller one, with a diameter of about one meter, and hop on exactly in the middle without shoes. Then you have to sway up and down, as if to take a leap into the air but without ever removing the soles of the feet from the structure.

You can do this exercise while watching TV by placing the mini-trampoline in front of the sofa; this small equipment is not difficult even to store when not in use, perhaps under the bed or across the side of a cabinet.

This exercise is known as "rebouncing", the simplest one but absolutely sufficient if practiced even just a couple of times a day for ten minutes at a time. On the Internet you can find many other ways to use the mini trampoline.

In addition, you could do this exercise outdoors: in those same 20 minutes, the sunlight would satisfy your daily vitamin D requirement and this simple aerobic exercise would also contribute to a better oxygenation of your Body tissues.

Please give me some more information on this topic of tissue oxygenation that you mentioned earlier, it seems very important to me. You told me that Dr. Warburg has reasonably attributed the beginning of cellular degeneration, which gives rise to tumors, precisely to a lack of oxygen that triggers a process in which the cells in order to survive begin to consume sugar instead of oxygen…

… well, in fact the cells always use sugar as an energy source but, when they don't have oxygen available to burn it in the chemical process called "breathing", they use 18 times as much in a process called "fermentation": one huge waste that generates the large amount of metabolic waste that initiates tissue degeneration.

I had never bothered to take enough oxygen.
Of course, I know I can stay weeks without eating and days without drinking but only a few minutes without breathing, but I never had a problem with it.
Indeed, now that I think about it, the idea that oxygenation is the secret in keeping the body healthy does not even surprise me a bit, after

all we are mainly composed of water which, in turn, is largely oxygen...

... and oxygen makes up 90% of the biological energy that allows the functioning of the body!

In fact, oxygen is not a targeted treatment for any disease but stimulates the Immune System and creates an inhospitable environment for pathogenic microorganisms.

In detail, I'm able to say that oxygen nourishes the cells, creates energy, fights fatigue, decomposes toxins and metabolic waste, brings the energy needed to assimilate the carbohydrates, regulates the pH of the Body, strengthens the defenses of Immune System and fights the invading organisms.

Therefore, all chronic-degenerative diseases can be countered by the administration of oxygen in adequate quantity, perhaps helping it to reach tissue cells with a vitamin supply: vitamin C facilitates the transport of oxygen in the cytoplasm and vitamin E through the cell membrane.

It's amazing the amount of things that I am learning in this conversation!

But how do I feed my Body's tissue cells with oxygen?

Is there a breathing technique to follow or should I inhale from an

oxygen tank?

I always consider useful breathing that fills the lungs as much as possible, not through the respiratory system though that you can think of sufficiently oxygenating the cells of your tissues to the point of reversing the degenerative process of your disease.

The so-called "oxidative biotherapies" involve the direct administration of oxygen, by absorbing it through the skin in a hyperbaric chamber, or the use of other compounds that release it easily.

It is used ozone, infused in the blood taken from the patient and then fed back into the circulation, and also hydrogen peroxide, intravenously or orally.

But hydrogen peroxide is oxygenated water! Are you advising me to drink hydrogen peroxide?

Listen, the hydrogen peroxide in the Body separates into water and oxygen.

The administration of hydrogen peroxide for therapeutic

use has been used successfully by over 10 million people in the last 170 years for about fifty different diseases.

It is the only administration of oxygen which does not require the support of a doctor and hydrogen peroxide also facilitates the release of oxygen by the hemoglobin.

You have to look for "food grade 35% hydrogen peroxide", because the one available in your pharmacy is only for external use; the protocol foresees the administration of an increasing number of drops and then decreasing it, always in a glass of distilled water, 3 times a day.

The therapy lasts about a month and a half and has a negligible cost, I tried it on myself to make sure it had no side effects and the only annoyance was not being able to eat before and after the intake of hydrogen peroxide to prevent it from reacting with food in the stomach, and thus damaging the walls.

You never stop to amaze me!
So could I recover from cancer by drinking hydrogen peroxide?

Mario, hydrogen peroxide is not an anticancer cure but it can slow down and even reverse the progressive degeneration of your Body's tissues: cancer cells don't like oxygen and the presence of oxygen in the tumor mass makes it even more sensitive to the effects of radiotherapy, allowing a reduction in exposure time.

In fact, it seems that part of the beneficial effect of vitamin C is because the it reacts with the copper present in the blood and producing its own hydrogen peroxide.

However, how is it possible that oxygen is not used by medical oncology?

Some clinics use ozone therapy but, in general, no Pharmaceutical Company has an interest in funding studies and investing resources in experiments on something that cannot produce any profit because it is not patentable.

I don't understand what surprises you, because to get a drug approved is very expensive, the procedure as a whole has a cost in the order of 150 million euros, and this protects the Pharmaceutical Industries because they can always accuse Alternative Medicine of using "drugs not approved" and making the public believe that this is synonymous with "unsafe" while the possibility of having a medicine approved is only an economic issue.

Today all oxidative biotherapies are considered

experimental and their use by doctors is forbidden, although over 6,000 articles on the subject are present in scientific literature.

After all, history remembers many doctors who administered oxygen to treat the most different diseases, where they empirically realized the existence of this "Life Force" which brings the Human Body back to Health but without ever having developed an interdisciplinary approach that could even do one prevention tool.

So would you suggest that I try drinking hydrogen peroxide?

Although oral use is controversial because oxygen is an oxidizing substance, I suggest it to anyone who has a chronic-degenerative disease and has not undergone transplants, in fact in the latter case by reinforcing the Immune System you risk the rejection of the organ transplanted.

Don't be so surprised, but hydrogen peroxide is present everywhere in Nature: both in rainwater and in Marian sources, as well as in breast milk (and even more in colostrum) in order to stimulate the infant's Immune System and to activate its metabolic processes. In your

Body it is produced by granulocytes to protect you from pathogens, it also regulates the thyroid functions and sex hormones.

However, as interesting as the subject is, we have spent too much time on it and I don't want you to get the idea that this is a sort of a "magic pill" because unfortunately it does not exist.

Now I have to talk to you about how to improve your mental approach to the disease.

You taught me many useful things to help my Body come back into balance.

I understand that much of this information is not of interest to the drug multinationals, but others may find some applications in the medical field.

How is it possible that there are no clinics with a different orientation?

There are, but they often had to be transferred to countries with a more tolerant legislation: for instance, almost all of those born in the US now operate in Mexico.

The fact is no doctor is allowed to treat patients on the basis of his discovery: even under the laws in force like Dr.

Stanislaw Burzynski, this researcher is still isolated in his clinic and opposed as much as possible. In fact, the results obtained by Burzynski have forced the FDA to approve his researches, but they are still not funded.

In addition, given the times that the law requires for experiments, things are not even better with regard to the methodologies now verified by different independent Institutes: the time necessary for the approval of a drug is between 10 and 20 years and it takes at least 15 years for the Medicine protocols to be updated with the latest Scientific discoveries.

Maybe you do not know, but most of the chemotherapy drugs in use today were approved 30 years ago!

Furthermore, history teaches that, even before legislating it, the inertia of Change requires that it takes a long time before the discoveries are reflected into practice: you must know it took several years after the discovery of the cause of the scurvy to become a habit bringing on vessels the vitamin C-rich citrus fruit!

And I thought I was being treated with cutting-edge techniques... the Truth is that I have to learn to take care of my Body like I have never done it before, but how I should have learned to do since I was a child.

Now I want to know everything about how to bring my Mind back into balance.

HOW TO BALANCE THE MIND

Very well, as usual before we go on I want to summarize in a few words the concepts related to the balance of the Body that we have talked about so far.

The Body is a wonderful machine, and you can abuse it for a long time before you get sick. The first cure will be to stop the incorrect behaviors and then help your Body to regain the balance by supplying it with important dosages of the nutrients that was before deprived and eliminating the substances that support the disease, in your case especially sugar and salt.

The keys of Body Wellbeing are a diet composed of almost exclusively vegetables consumed raw and very moderate in quantity, to give the organism then the possibility of purifying itself, a bit of physical activity and sufficient time spent outdoors.

And that's all.

Vegetables in salad, no salt, carrot juice, I will not enjoy eating that!

Your philosophy could be summed up in this way, saying "God made the food and the Devil the kitchen", but when can I go back to eating normally?

If you were to return to the diet that started the cancer, you would most likely get sick again.

Over time, you will refine the taste for this "divine" diet and you will find everything that you thought desirable to be indigestible, you just have to follow my instructions patiently without expecting to not have to make an effort.

The work you will do with the Mind will help you, a necessary job because you need to know that the mentality with which you face disease is even more important than diet.

The Mind plays a fundamental symbolic role in developing this disease and has the same Power even in the Healing process.

I remember blushing as a result of certain emotions and, in general, it is not difficult for me to accept the fact that the Thoughts Patterns produce effects on the physical Body because I imagine that the brain biochemically is connected to the Body and therefore in some way able to control it. Nevertheless, I don't have the tools to make the Mind work in my favor.

I feel stressed by Life, full of thoughts, at the mercy of my emotions...

This is the reason why I often find useful in cases like yours that you get support from a Counselor capable and open to the issues covered in this dialogue.

However, this is not absolutely necessary, as there are several psychological self-help tools that can support you as you redefine the way your Mind sees the World.

I am not at all surprised by how you describe yourself and I assure you that you are in good company: almost all of my patients feel stressed even if objectively they shouldn't be, or at least they could not be.

The definition of illness as an "unprocessed stressful experience" refers however only to the emotional aspect, while I prefer to place it within a broader context that includes its expression in the physical Body, of which we have already spoken, and its spiritual causes, of which we will talk.

Ok, stress is an emotional contributory cause of cancer.

This is what Walter told me when he read Norman Cousins'
psychoneuroimmunology: it seems to be definitively proven that stress
inhibits the Immune System.
I would like instead to understand from you how "I could" be less
stressed with the Life I conduct, to be more calm I should distance
myself from my problems and above all from several people I am
forced to work with.

You are wrong again, I have already explained to you that
your stress does not depend on external circumstances but
on the Perception you have on them and the Perception is
the filter you have before your eyes and is under the control
of your Belief System.

Ultimately, we could say that cancer is the reflection of a
Belief System that no longer supports the Body.

The simplest explanation is the scenario in which the
disease develops because unconsciously we see death as the
only possible solution to a situation that otherwise we
believe not to be able to manage.

You talked to me about the techniques of Energetic Psychology able to
rewrite the Beliefs deposited in my Unconscious, first of all by
practicing EFT.

On the Internet, you will find a lot of material, look for the right tool for you: if you don't find yourself at ease with EFT, you can try the BSFF or the Psych-K.

They are all tools where you can learn to manage your Beliefs and consequently live all the emotions peacefully and without becoming a chronic and boring thing.

By intervening on the Belief System, you will find yourself thinking differently and... well, did I mention to you that the Reality around us is determined by Thoughts, Words and Works?

Yes, you were telling me, I was watching you with some suspicion, but now I'm a little more inclined to listen to you.

There is a beautiful phrase of the Buddha that says: "All that we are is the result of what we have thought".

This means that you are the Law that regulates your World, I read it in a book by Dr. John Randolph Price.

The ancient Alchemists would have said that Isis listens to recurring thoughts during your day and defines your mental state accordingly, and then uses his Creative Power to manifest this state outside through the events of your Life.

Creating is an inner work during which we consciously pay

attention to a possibility that already exists.

In other words: you will experience events that are in tune with what you think about most often, because you are what you frequently think about all day long.

It is what sustains the Law of Attraction explained in another way: my thoughts attract in my Life events that are similar to what I am thinking and therefore the most effective strategy to make happen what I wish is that I expect it so, quite sure the Universe is already preparing it for me.

Exactly, the problem is that most people do not recognize that they have this Creative Power and they create at random by constantly changing their focus: they focus on something but, not having the patience to wait for their manifestation in the physical world, they soon start thinking of other things.

In alchemical terms, we could say that in this way, they let the Male Principle of others fertilize the receptivity of their Female Principle.

Wait George, I could accept that my Mind had control over my Body through the endocrine system, but now you're suggesting that I can also influence events in the World out there, just through the perception that I have of them?

I would like to give you this Belief because it would make you leap forward, but it is not necessary for your Change on the road to Healing.

However, if you succeeded in making this your idea, you would accept everything you thought you had to fight with, including the illness, because you would recognize it as a mere projection of your unconsciousness.

Your relationships will also benefit because, instead of condemning others, you would recognize that they are only mirrors that are showing you certain parts of you that you do not love and that are an extraordinary opportunity to observe yourself and solve your problems, and to see them dissolve even in others.

It is an extremely empowering vision of yourself and of the World.

I believe it but, for now, it is beyond the possibilities of my Mind.
I studied some quantum physics and I read the experiments that show a sort of inexplicable connection between particles, the so-called "entanglement»", but I still struggle to accept that even people and

things are connected to each other, to the point that the Reality around me depends on what I think.

I understand, it is a way of seeing things that gives me a lot of Power but I cannot believe it.

As I explained to you, it is not necessary even if you have to know that Indian Ayurvedic Medicine already taught that consciousness generates matter.

You can still think of working with EFT to modify your Belief System to remain open to the possibility that things are this way.

Think about it, you're just giving up one limiting scheme.

Because I think your skeptical rationality can be helped by a concrete case, I will tell you the Ho'oponopono: a simple and at the same time extraordinary technique, which works right on the principle of mutual connection between people.

It was developed by the shamans of the Hawaiian Islands and is based on the concept that the problems are not the places, the situations and the people around us, but the thoughts we have about them: the problems are only "painful memories that come back", personal or borrowed from the collective Beliefs that sustain them in the World.

The approach of the Ho'oponopono is therefore to limit itself to noticing the problem and to ask God, renouncing to every control, to neutralize the energy field in us that we associate with that person, that place or that thing.

It has a lot to do with "allowing" something to happen rather than "trying to make it happen".

This is done by repeating 4 magic phrases: "I love you, I'm sorry, May you forgive me, Thank you" addressed precisely to God within us: we choose, but we entrust ourselves completely to God who knows what is best for us. Practically we cancel the limits of intentionality.

Of all the amazing things that you told me, this is the weirdest one! The ancient Hawaiians who utter 4 magical phrases should help me rationally accept the existence of a connection between all people?

The example I'm doing to you is very relevant to what we were talking about, because through the Ho'oponopono you clean up the Belief within you that has manifested the problem that others are showing you, now I get to the reason why all this proves a connection between people.

Years ago a psychologist, Dr. Ihaleakala Hew Len, was placed by the Hawaiian government at the head of the island's mental hospital and resolved many of the most difficult cases without ever even meeting the patients but by just pronouncing these sentences in front of their medical records: he was assuming full responsibility for the situation in which the sick were suffering because they had become part of his experience of Life and therefore their Healing depended on his thoughts.

And do you expect me to believe this story? How can I have proof that it is true?

Mario, I read it on a very pleasant book by Joe Vitale and I found confirmation from other sources but I don't expect you to believe it, nor will I try to convince you of its truth.

Your rationality would never allow you to believe in it completely even if you were to take a plane to Hawaii and manage to access the hospital's archives, first you need to make room for events like this in your Belief System.

Someone had said that Faith of the size of a mustard seed is enough for everything to become possible, I am telling you that you can earn that Faith by rewriting the Belief Patterns in your Unconscious and that this process is not difficult but, simply using the appropriate tools, it just takes time and determination.

It is written, "You will receive according to your Faith."
I don't know what to tell you, George.
Perhaps you are right, it may be true that over time I will change
slowly and I will also be able to accept what today seems incredible to
me.
However, where do you advise me to start?

Experiment, experiment, experiment. Become a researcher.
To listen to me without putting into practice what I say is
like to stay thirsty looking at a glass of water instead of
drinking it. It serves no purpose!
Try EFT and the Ho'oponopono, try to say the phrase "I
accept myself unconditionally right now" looking at
yourself in the mirror, and do that useful exercise of
looking at a beautiful smiling photo of your past for 30
seconds and then close your eyes and imagine yourself in
that happy Body.
You can also start with the simpler Positive Thinking
introduced by Louise Hay: fill the home, office and car with
positive thoughts so that, by rereading them, you can slowly
change. The Unconscious is written with a patient

repetition.

Do you want some very powerful advice? Dare to start the reminder sentences with "I am..." and then always talk in the present time: don't write, "so be it", instead write "so it is".

Maybe "I am Healed", what do you say?
Just thinking about it, I seem to write a lie!

If this is the feeling you feel writing that sentence, it simply means that you are not yet ready to write it and that, unfortunately, you are not yet going in that direction.

Always keep in mind the words of Neville Goddard: "You do not attract what you want, but what you believe to be true" or, if you prefer, the even more demanding version of Dr. Wayne Dyer: "You don't attract what you want, you attract what you are".

I personally find this concept extraordinarily expressed in the words of Master Sri Nisargadatta Maharaj "Things do not happen because I make them happen but because I am", they make the idea that in order to experience something we must "be" that thing through an act of will and that consequently the human being becomes what he believes to be.

You can start with an annotation such as "I am on the road to Healing" which may be acceptable to you and which cannot even be contradicted by a possible result of a clinical examination that is not exactly in line with your wishes.

The idea is that you have already obtained what you want at the very moment you ask for and that you just have to wait for it to appear on the physical plane, you have only to put yourself in the position to be prepared to receive it.

Remember that you choose what you want by inserting yourself in the divine flow and leave it to God to create what is best for you, to then accept any result without attachment to your initial choice.

And everything should be done always, always, always with an extreme Gratitude.

Here you invent something new, I learned to recognize that look when you raise your eyes and stare at me as if you had said something very important.

I 'm listening to you, tell me about Gratitude.

It is one of the most fundamental keys to the success of

mental work: you must prove Gratitude for having received what is best for you and you must do it the moment you ask, before seeing any results.

You are asking me something impossible: Gratitude is proved in the face of having been satisfied and I am not healed, I cannot feel it beforehand!
And anyway, I'm not able to feel these emotions on command.

You will have to learn, I have already explained to you that by changing what you experience can change things.

Mental techniques can help you to find a justification for what you decide to feel emotionally; I remember a seminar by the Hicks couple who encouraged a sort of dialogue between themselves aimed at finding motivations for the state of mind that was chosen in advance.

Experience Gratitude because at this precise moment an irreversible process of Healing has started within your Body, experience Gratitude because God has given you an extraordinary opportunity for growth through this disease, experience Gratitude for having discovered that you are responsible for your Health, experience Gratitude because today is the first day of your New Life.

As you can see you do not need an event to be grateful, it is enough that you want it.

I personally think that "being grateful" is one of the inevitable verbs beyond a certain level of personal growth, along with others such as "to love", "to forgive", "to thank", "to bless", "to honor", "to consecrate" and "to celebrate".

And, if it is true that our experiences determine our emotional state and our thoughts, now I teach you an extraordinary technique: to correct your memories.

The basic idea is to erase an unpleasant memory by inventing one of imagination and replacing it into one's memory: in the evening review your day by rewriting the encounters and dialogues you experienced but of which you are not satisfied, correct them as you wish and relive them at your own pace in the smallest emotional details.

Have people tell you what you want them to say to you and then go beyond, by writing to you alone letters with the words you would like to receive from them... in a short time others will testify with their actions about the Change that happened inside of you, and the different ways they appear in your eyes!

Do you mean that if I take care to build in details invented memories, it will be like having lived them?

You absolutely must try an exercise that Rhonda Byrne suggests in one of her books: write the list of your ten most beautiful wishes as if they had already come true, that is, in the form "Thank you, thank you, thank you for..." and follow the wish!

Then, for each one, answer these three questions: "What emotions did you feel when your wish come true?", "To whom did you tell it first and how did you tell it?", "What was the first thing you did as soon as you made your wish?".

In fact, these questions lead you ingeniously to live your desire as if had already come true, both emotionally and from a sensory point of view.

I still remember how well I feel after doing this exercise, it was a significant experience that I will hardly forget.

I can't believe it!

Not only you can, but also you must; because it suits you.

Freeing your Mind from the limits that do not allow you to

believe this kind of things, allows you to enter a fantastic World, at your disposal if you just stop giving it up.

A World in which visualization is a therapeutic tool because you can "see" your Body's systems returning to balance and you can help your Immune System simply by imagining it attacking and destroying the weak tumor cells.

In principle, the visualization is able to support all the defense mechanisms of the Body identified by Dr. Josef Issels: the Immune System of lymphocytes and antibodies, the detoxification organs (intestine, skin, kidneys and liver), the epithelial tissue bacteria that cover the body cavities and the connective tissue that eliminates toxins and harmful microorganisms.

These techniques have been practiced successfully for decades even in psychodynamics.

Listen, the concept of "spontaneous remission" must be explained, it requires a cause: all cases of spontaneous remission occur in patients with a positive attitude and this has led to the development of mental and visualization techniques.

That's all, for a more structured approach, you can read books by Dr. Carl Simonton or you can attend one of his seminars where you will learn the importance of doing what you like and the benefits that this brings to your Body-Mind System, as the Psycho-Neuro-Endocrine-Immunology (PNEI) teaches.

Remember that the point is not what a vision should be but all that it can do, that's the only thing that matters.

The list of names I'm writing down is getting longer and I think you still need to talk about how to balance the Spirit, I'm listening.

HOW TO BALANCE THE SPIRIT

Trusting that you no longer have any doubts about the Power that your Mind can exercise on your Body and that you are also willing to consider the effects of your thought on the events of your Life, I now want to talk to you about Meditation and Prayer.

Walter explained to me that Meditation is the detoxification of the Mind and it is very useful to release the stress that weakens the Immune System.

I totally agree with Walter, but now I would like to take you a little further, reconnecting to what I told you before, and inviting you to a meditation state in which you prepare your future with the Mind and then let go of all the resistance, and by trusting yourself that what you wish already exists and should not be "made it happen" in any way.

But even the Meditation is a mental technique such as those that you have described to me so far!

I don't have to believe in the existence of the Spirit...

This is a way of seeing things, overall is the least interesting one.

In fact, I would like you to take advantage of the meditation state precisely to distance yourself from your Mind, understood as Ego, Personality, and reach a sort of "Connection with your Higher Self, with God".

The Ego is a result of our Life experiences that make us believe that we are what we have, what we do and what others think of us... and these ideas are the basis of our daily patterns!

Each of us instead is a sacred divine spark through which God experiences himself but, by answering your question, you can do without believing in all this and limit yourself to using Meditation and Prayer as techniques aimed at fulfilling your desires.

If today you are at this point in your personal Life journey, I will limit myself to saying this, certain that it will be the practice to allow you a deeper understanding of what you were doing: an action to rebalance your spiritual energy.

Thank you for not expecting too much from me, give me some guidance on how to practice Meditation in the simplest way possible so that I can benefit from it without having to believe that I have God within me!

All right, the day will come when you will want to know something more.

I advise you to use the Vipassana Meditation, which aims to develop maximum attention to all sensory and mental stimulation. I invite you to start with two exercises that highlight how your awareness is outside of your Mind: in the first you simply have to observe your breath without changing it and, in the second, waiting for the first thought that comes to your Mind and recognize it.

The difficulty is not to practice for a few seconds but to do it for about twenty minutes: soon you will no longer have control of yourself and your head will be lost behind something. Do not worry and do not condemn yourself for something that is absolutely normal, but instead gently return to the exercise by letting go of the thought that distracted you.

That's all?

And what should I expect after having devoted twenty minutes a day to these exercises?

The goal is to reach a greater state of "Presence", the awareness that Life is now and that this is the only Reality, while we usually suffer from a Past that is no longer and worrying about a Future that most of the times will never be.

If you think about it, much of the suffering that comes from an event is experienced just by rethinking it and, similarly, the concern for a feared future is often worse even than the moment in which you had to experience that eventuality.

You absolutely must read the works of Eckhart Tolle.

I remember an example in which he invited people to consciously live every moment of their daily lives, even during those moments when they brought a glass of water to their mouths, without wanting to be at the moment when their lips would have rested on the edge of the glass.

And by practicing Meditation could I get to develop this vigilant attention that allows me to realize that in the present moment, there is no problem but simply my existence?

Exactly. The well-known "I Am", so ineffable that it can be defined only by exclusion: "You are what remains when you have excluded all that you are not".

It is interesting, but I have the idea that the control of one's Mind requires a hard training of many years, I imagine the long sessions of the Tibetan monks in search of Illumination...

The Mind works by associations and continually jumps from one thought to another like a monkey.

Turning off the "mental chatter" requires a greater effort than your own abilities, limit yourself observing the Mind in its way of thinking and then image the thoughts that you have made like balloons, will you let them go until you see them lost in the sky, or like boats that move away on the horizon until they disappear.

Replace the effort with the gentle letting go but, above all, get out of your head that Enlightenment is a state to be reached with a very long training; this kind of ideas greatly gratify the Mind but postpone the achievement of the goal by focusing on intermediate steps that do not exist: Enlightenment is available Here and Now, renouncing the anticipation that gives insecurity and the memory that brings unhappiness.

George, I really start to struggle to follow you even if, observing anything around me, I realize how many memories I associate with them... I understand that the goal is to look at the World for what it is, "becoming a child", that is before the Mind collected all those categories it uses to filter the information it receives from the senses.

Very well, I will follow your instructions on Meditation and I will make this experience.

But now tell me something about Prayer, I have always been fascinated by Mark 9:23 who says, "All things are possible to him who believes".

If you have read the Gospel of Mark, in Chapter 11:24 it also offers you the formula to get everything you want: "Therefore I say to you, whatever you ask with Prayers, believe that you have already received it and you will get it".

It seems to me to be aligned with what I have already told you when talking about mental techniques, what do you think?

In fact, Gregg Braden treats Prayer just like a technique and calls it the "forgotten technology of Prayer".

Precisely in this sense, he recalls that Prayer has nothing to do with the daily murmur of most people, as it is not an act of will in which you implore God to realize your own desires, it's a matter of recognizing oneself as being what you want.

Beautiful words, but how do you suggest me to begin this practice?

Start by using the powerful state of drowsiness that precedes sleep, in order to prolong all night long the feelings of satisfaction that I invite you to try, and see yourself gratified by the realization of your desires.

Don't imagine yourself from the outside, as if you were seeing yourself in a film, but from inside your Body with all the richness of the sensory stimulation of the environment that surrounds you: look at the shapes and colors, listen to the sounds, and appreciate the sense of touch... but above all emotionally test what you would experience if everything had already gone as you wish, Here and Now.

Remember to keep a burning and focused thought, focused in one direction, that your Mind must be dominated by that one feeling, which is the realization of your desire.

So the feeling is the secret for a prayer to be heard, it is the leavening that allows the exercise of one's Creative Power.

In practice, I should discipline myself in order to experience only the feelings that contribute to my happiness, to observe my thoughts and to choose with what to nourish my Mind, instead of being a victim of the usual mental automatism.

Now I finally understand the sense of the Meditation exercise you explained to me a little while ago...

An uncritical observation of that internal dialogue that incessantly talks in our heads also reveals to us the Beliefs through which we see the World, we could say that this dialogue literally manifests itself in what happens around us.

Mario, you can do Miracles by keeping control of your thoughts without condemning them and replacing the usual internal mechanical dialogue with a Conscious one, based on the feeling that your desires have been satisfied.

Okay, you've opened a door in front of me but I don't know if I'm ready to venture out.

Listen, George, we talked for a long time and I learned many things, most of which I reserve the right to check out and investigate, but if our roles were reversed and you were on this side of the desk, what would you do to enhance this dialogue with the practice?

HAVE A NICE TRIP

I would accept the challenge and undertake my personal Healing Journey, at all levels, supported by the Truth that suggest these simple evangelical words: "Your Bodies become what you eat, just as your thoughts become Your Spirit".

From the time I spent talking, I would try to take home a little more of what I'm ready to accept right now, like when an athlete tries to do a little more than he knows he can do.

You know Mario, I believe in everything I told you but, in good faith, I might have been wrong about something or I might have even given you information not suitable for you right now.

In any case, I urge you not to "throw away the baby together with the bathwater" and remain open to every possibility, even to those that today may seem incredible to you.

How can you be so indifferent to the fact that something is true or false?

Listening to you talk it seems that for you it is not so bad to believe and base your decisions on something that one day may prove to be wrong.

The same Science, which you so much esteem, is a succession of theories that are periodically changed: first the World is flat and then spherical, first the Sun revolves around the Earth and then vice versa... is this a cause for scandal?

I prefer to see the Truth from the point of view of its usefulness: every Truth no longer functional naturally becomes the humus in which it takes root and from which a subsequent higher Truth is nourished.

And this is a very individual process in which it is inappropriate to interfere.

But you explained to me things that radically changed my way of seeing the World, you interfered heavily in what I can define as "my Truth about the World".

You taught me that the diagnosis of a disease can be the beginning of a long learning process in which the choice to survive is an experience of conversion to the depth of Life.

I am part of your World, and since Fate does not exist, my role in your Life could not be different from what it was.

Moreover, I am with the idea of letting everyone experience their own Truth and reap the benefits, in order to evolve at their own pace without being intellectually attacked by anyone else in that sort of mental war that is the attempt to convince you.

I like to consider myself "at your service", as every human being should be for the rest of Humanity.

For me, sharing what I believe is a way of experiencing what I am through my expression; this is the main sense of "giving", opposed to the madness of "must become" characteristic of the Ego.

So let me ask you once again what I should do when I get out of your office.

What is the most important thing that I should remember?

I could fill you with good advice, reminding you to see anyone with Gratitude and to multiply the interpersonal relationships you find pleasant, but also suggesting that you predigest the raw and nutritious food with few calories-sugar-fat-proteins and by chewing it until it becomes liquid, reactivating your circulation with moments of cold water during a hot shower and often rubbing your body with a towel... but I want you to not forget the most important thing: winning cancer is a decision and you have to decide, because every patient has the best doctor within himself.

And in your decisions, I advise you first of all to be "a good animal" giving priority to what makes you feel good.

Minimize the medical treatment, supporting it with positive thoughts and good nutrition and... make long-term plans for your future!

No, wait. Please explain.

What do you mean by "minimizing medical treatment"?

It seemed to me that you was against chemotherapy because it only reduces the tumor mass, which is only a symptom of cancer, and, at the same time, aggravates the intoxication and therefore the imbalance of the Body.

And what about long-term plans?

You remember exactly what I told you: tumors are just the manifestations of cancer and Paracelsus was right in arguing that eliminating the disease symptoms is like wiping the snow from the front door in an attempt to ward off winter.

However, I also explained to you that in some cases a tumor mass can be dangerous and that the large amount of degenerated cells contribute to keeping the organism in a state of imbalance.

These are the reasons why I do not exclude the utility of surgery, chemotherapy and radiotherapy, but I suggest a responsible and conscious use of it, and only after understanding the importance of food and mental hygiene, as well as the physical exercise.

As for long-term plans... well, it's just a ploy to make sure that your Mind doesn't even consider the possibility of not being there in a few years!

For example, you could say to yourself: "I must be around to be present at my son's graduation!"

We have talked at length about the Power of the Unconscious, in practice you get the exact opposite effect to when a colleague of mine tells you that you have 6 months of Life left.

However, remember that cancer is not a death sentence:

you can heal completely and also live with it for a very long time with an excellent quality of Life, it is only a matter of supporting the Body's self-Healing abilities, always bearing in mind that patience is the only assistant of Mother Nature.

Yes, yes, but I still feel so ignorant and I don't feel like taking the Responsibility of my Health to the point of contradicting your colleagues.

You keep talking about common sense but with common sense I don't find answers to everything.

I give you an example: over the summer, I like to drink very cold water, does it hurt? How can I understand it with common sense without the knowledge of the human Body that a doctor has?

What do you think a doctor knows more about you with the example you did?

I also think only with common sense.

It is known that when two bodies of different temperatures are put in contact, after a while they reach the same temperature: if you remove butter from the refrigerator and place it on the table, after a while it will warm up.

Well, similarly if I eat or drink anything at a different

temperature than my Body, my Body will have to do a job to bring this food to the Body temperature.

This is the only thing that happens and you could understand it by yourself: when you drink cold water, and force your body to heat it up by consuming some of your Body's resources.

It is therefore better not to do so, especially in your case because you are already weakened.

Now you also understand the reason for the congestion: a thermal shock following a big job that you requested from your Body, which failed to manage with available resources.

Everything has a simple explanation, often accessible with common sense and without any specific knowledge.

Often, but not always.

No, not always.

In fact, in a case as delicate as yours, I recommend a team of supportive people who work on nutrition, food supplementation, detoxification and exercise.

Surround yourself with positive people and therapists who develop your independence and are not afraid to contradict the medical class: they continually contradict each other without even giving you their excuses.

I remember TV commercials from a few decades ago in which American doctors were advertising Philip Morris cigarettes, by smoking in a white coat in their office.

Today even patients are not allowed to smoke in the doctor's office, and in the future I expect that doctors will be forbidden to keep attitudes harmful to Health, even in private Life.

In fact, a smoker and overweight doctor who professes "Do what I say and not as I do" conveys an ambiguous and inconsistent message to his patient.

Now I also realize how important it is for the patient to choose their doctor: aware of his ignorance, he feels the need to put his trust in someone he trusts completely.

It is your right to question everything you are told by me and by my colleagues, especially when faced with contradictory behavior; I read about a survey that showed that 70% of oncologists would not undergo chemotherapy, nor will they recommend it to a relative.

It is a situation similar to that of a financial advisor who finds himself selling insurance products that he himself would not buy.

Find out about the success of the treatment that is offered to you for your specific illness in the hospital that is treating you, you owe it to yourself and to the people who care about your Health.

Don't be ashamed to ask and become suspicious in the face of an elusive or even aggressive response: we doctors often react by showing ourselves upset by not answering a question that would highlight our ignorance in Alternative Therapies and even unprepared for what we are proposing. We fear that the patient who wants to know what is being administered to him, because we do not know exactly what we are doing and are afraid he may notice it.

You're teaching me to be wary of doctors as I am of my insurance company!

It depends on the meaning you attribute to the term "to be wary"

I think that all doctors act in good faith, when they consider doing their job as a cog in a more complex mechanism.

Unfortunately, however, they can operate limitedly to the

indications received from the Ministry of Health, which is strongly conditioned by the economic interests of Pharmaceutical Companies.

In this way, doctors lack the overview that would allow them to understand the causes of illness; the one according to which the disease is born in the Mind and only later manifests itself in the Body, all according to the plans of the Spirit.

I am inviting you to ask yourself, together with your doctor, about the costs and benefits of each therapy offers to you. Just this one.

Yeah, you're good at saying "just this one", but it's not easy for me. Sometimes it seems that you forget that, since I found out I was sick, I am experiencing in a moment of deep crisis.

In the Chinese language, the term "crisis" is written using two distinct ideograms, the first meaning "danger" and the second "opportunity".

Passing by this disease, you have the greatest opportunity to see Life in a different way; many cancer patients claim that cancer was the greatest teaching they could benefit from in order to change their Lifestyle and, transformed it into an opportunity for personal growth, they defined it as the best thing that ever happened to them and to the family and to the friends who shared the experience.

Cancer can heal Life by teaching you to understand it, through Responsibility and Gratitude for everything we live.

Remember that experience is not what happens to you but what you do as a result of what happens to you.

It is an alarm for change and not a punishment.
While you were talking to me, right now, I caught a sort of Perfection in this disease.
For a moment, I could have called it "appropriate for me right now."
I know it may sound silly, but I would use the term "Miracle".

Everything in Life is a Miracle for those who believe in it, nothing is for those who do not believe it.

You just have to choose which side you are on and consequently live the Life you have chosen.

I learned a game that I practice whenever I remember it during the day: I simply say to myself, "Isn't it wonderful?" by taking care to suspend the rationality, which immediately asks what on earth is referring to something so wonderful.

The goal is to slowly change my Perception of the World using a filter that makes me see everything as wonderful and everything takes on the appearance of a Miracle in my eyes.

The poet Kahlil Gibran wrote, "The way we see things depends on our state of mind and when we see Magic and Beauty in them, in reality they are in us".

Mario, I know that believing everything I told you is scary because our community does not support those who do not submit to its rules, but if you do not begin to manage your Reality, you will be left at the mercy of it.

I gave you new eyes to see the World and it's a great World to live in.

Believe me.

I believe you, George.
I believe you.

REFERENCE AUTHORS

During the dialogue were mentioned several Authors: they are listed below in alphabetical order for the convenience of the reader interested in further investigations.

Athias, Gérard

Beard, John

Braden, Gregg

Budwig, Johanna

Burzynski, Stanislaw

Buteyko, Konstantin

Byrne, Rhonda

Caisse, René

Campbell, Colin

Clark, Hulda

Cousins, Norman

Craig, Gary

Dwoskin, Hale

Dyer, Wayne

Ehret, Arnold

Gerson, Max e Charlotte

Gibran, Kahlil

Griffin, Edward

Goddard, Neville

Hamer, Ryke Geerd

Hay, Louise

Hellinger, Bert

Hew Len, Ihaleakala

Hicks, Esther e Jerry

Hoxsey, Harry

Howell, Edward

Issels, Josef

Jung, Carl Gustav

Kelley, William Donald

Krebs, Ernest

Lammers, Willem

Lipton, Bruce

Livingston, Virginia

Maharaj, Nisargadatta

Mereu, Gabriella

Nims, Larry

Pasteur, Louis

Pauling, Linus

Price, John Randolph

Rainville, Claudia

Rife, Royal Raymond

Schützenberger, Anne Ancelin

Simoncini, Tullio

Simonton, Carl

Tolle, Eckhart

Vitale, Joe

Walsch, Neale Donald

Warburg, Otto

Young, Robert

Zeland, Vadim

(Written between summer and autumn 2012)

www.ingramcontent.com/pod-product-compliance
Lightning Source LLC
Chambersburg PA
CBHW062200280526
45788CB00001B/377